Taming the MG Dragon

Journey through a myasthenic crisis

One woman's story of her life threatening experience and recovery from Myasthenia Gravis, an Auto-immune disease 2016.

Taming the MG Dragon

Journey through a Myasthenic Crisis

*One woman's story of her life threatening experience
and recovery from Myasthenia Gravis,
an Auto-immune disease 2016*

Mereti Taipana-Howe

Taming the MG Dragon:*Journey through a Myasthenic Crisis* published by Rangitawa Publishing, Feilding, New Zealand. 2017

ISBN 978-0-9941490-0-8

www.rangitawapublishing.com
rangitawa@xtra.co.nz

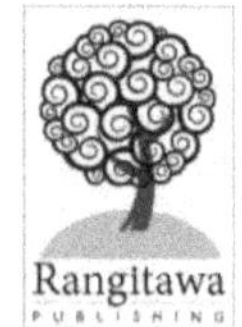

Contents

PART 1 THE MG DRAGON

Myasthenia Gravis – life-threatening crisis

'To me a dragon is magnificent, tyrannical, and deadly. One has got to learn all about the dragon and how to ride it, to tame it.'

PART 2   TAMING THE MG DRAGON

Specialist Rehabilitation services within the hospital (1)

'I think one of the main goals of the ICU staff was to be able to discharge patients from the ICU and move them towards rehabilitation, because it meant the person was through the worst of their ordeal and on their way home. Seeing a person move forward in their recovery is a highlight, and a reward for all of their (and the patient's) hard work.'

Specialist Rehabilitation services within the hospital (2)

'For me, as a Maori patient, the Whare Rapuora Unit

means that the cultural needs of the Tangata Whenua are acknowledged and respected. Whare Rapuora staff are specialists, not only providing cultural consultancy to the DHB, carrying out Powhiri and other cultural protocols for the hospital, but also assisting patients in the areas of social work, advocacy, and cultural needs in all wards of the hospital. Culture is important. New Zealand is now more culturally diverse than ever before.'

PART 3. POST-HOSPITAL RECOVERY

<u>Chapter 21</u>
After 5 months, it's home time!   111

'My self-care is now down to me. I don't see myself as an invalid and if I want to reclaim my independence, then as much as possible it's up to me to pave my own way. I've definitely adopted the 'Whare Tapa Wha' care model to guide me through. This involves care of the physical, the mental health and aspirations, whānau and relationships, and the spiritual aspects of a person.'

<u>Chapter 22</u>
Through my family's eyes   116

Families and friends of loved ones in hospital go through their own ordeal as they try to come to terms with the changes that serious illness makes to their lives. I think it was best described as 'nga piki me nga heke' by my younger brother, and that's what supporters go through: a rollercoaster ride, emotionally, and psychologically, especially the children and immediate whānau of the

FOREWORD

Tena koutou.

This book is about the impacts of Myasthenia Gravis. It provides vivid accounts of the illness and the accompanying crises that create serious risks for recovery, if not for life. Because the disease is relatively rare, the insights contained in *'Taming the MG Dragon'* will be important to understanding the illness and dealing with the complications. In that respect, it will have particular significance for neurologists, intensive care physicians and nurses, physiotherapists, social workers and rehabilitation experts in New Zealand, but across the wider global health network as well.

While the focus has been on Myasthenia Gravis, this book is also about human resilience, faith, courage and bravery. Mereti speaks from the heart and insofar as she delves into her own dark moments, she speaks much more loudly about her commitment to life and her resolve to overcome what must have appeared to be relentless odds. Much more than a documentation of events, she has provided a very personal account of the ways in which she coped when she was unable to speak, unable to move freely, unable to control her own muscles, unable to eat or breathe on her own, and unable to make her own views known. Writing was to become an important vehicle for making sense of the whole experience and then sharing it with others.

Many people suffer unexpected health crises that require lengthy treatment and care, often accompanied by a sense of despair and the loss of hope. *'Taming the MG Dragon'* is testament to the power of recovery and to the strength of tenacity. Much of that strength came from Mereti herself and from exemplary health care but whānau and friends were also to become critical links with the world beyond the hospital. By bringing that world to the bedside, there was an opportunity for her to live in it, largely through the eyes and ears of others, but nonetheless sufficient to generate an absolute determination to go home.

Across the chapters in this book, are lessons for all of us but the obvious conclusion must be that dragons don't win.

Kia ora.

Mason Durie KNZM

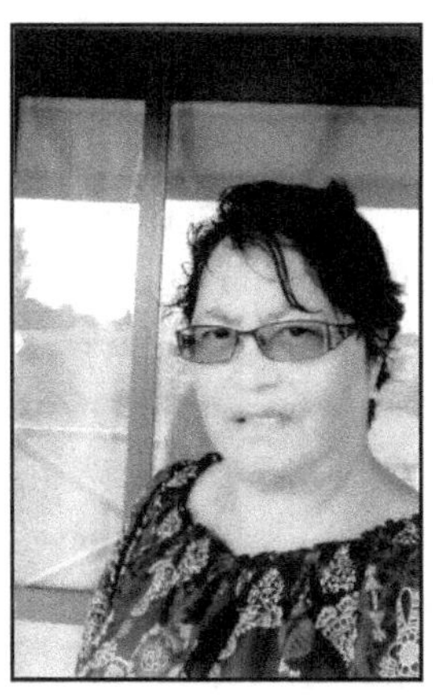

About the Author

Mereti is from Aotearoa/New Zealand. She has worked in the disability sector as a NASC (Needs Assessor Service Coordinator) in government departments and tertiary institutions as an adult tutor. Mereti was educated at a private Maori school, Turakina Maori Girls College (Marton). In later life she completed and graduated from Auckland University with an Advanced Certificate in Conflict Resolution, and from Massey University with two Social Science Degrees and a post-graduate Diploma in Disability Studies within the health sector. In addition to university training, she underwent specific training in the counselling field at the Human Development and Training Institute of NZ and Wellington Institute of Technology.

In 2008, she established her own counselling consultancy, providing counselling in a vast range of topics: Cultural Consultancy, Clinical and Professional Supervision, and Training.

Mereti is descended from the indigenous people of Aotearoa (Maori or Tangata Whenua). Her tribes are: Ngati Kauwhata, Rangitane, Rangatahi, and Ngati Toa on her mother's side, and Kaati Mamoe, Kai Tahu on her father's side. She currently lives in the Manawatu.

Illness from Myasthenia Gravis (MG) has impacted greatly on her life, and while it is important to pace her activities and days at the time of writing this, she continues to stay connected to the things that matter most to her: whānau, iwi, marae, mahi, and hapori. In this book, she tells her story in the hope that it will help others with this condition, and in one way or another provide a platform for anyone working with MG sufferers.

Acknowledgements

I would like to acknowledge my whānau. My brothers Charles, Tiratahi and Maui, my sister Hurihia, my sister in law Sandy, my daughter Ngaio and Sandra,Rachel, Raewyn, and team from Totara Trust. My son Te Whiu (Tef), who has been there for me since I got home. My cousins, nieces and nephews who always called in to visit me in hospital, even when they were visiting from afar. Knowing my whānau were there kept me strong.

Those who lived close regularly called in to see how I was, and updated me on our marae and whanui activities. A special perfume from whānau Arohia and Mason, takes pride of place on my dressing table.
This beautiful perfume forever reminds me of my recovery and rejuvenation time. The special and enlightening korero we had during each visit kept me positive. Whānau is a pou of strength.

Thank you to the friends and colleagues who made phone calls on my behalf and helped me with work matters; to those who sent cards, texts and emails to ICU; to those special people I had worked with, who came in especially to see me.

Lastly, thank you to the people from the Kaumatua ukulele group of Whare Rapuora (Maori

14

Health Unit) who visited and played music to me during my recovery in the ICU and in the rehabilitation ward. I felt so spoilt.

Knowing the busy lives everyone had, I'm grateful that they visited and kept me in their thoughts.

I acknowledge the medical professionals who, with their special kind of weaponry, helped me fight the MG dragon and get back to my life. There are too many to mention all of them by name, but they are the doctors, consultants and nurses who looked after me during my hospital stay. Special acknowledgement to Dr Daniel Nistor, Head Consultant, and Charge Nurse Sue Kirkman; Dr Rau Fu, and many others of the Intensive Care Unit (ICU), and the Star 2 Jaimee; my Social Worker in the rehab ward, Telesia; my Occupational Therapist Jody and her assistant Cherine; Neurology Consultant Dr P. Carigas, and Drs I and M Rodrigues; Registrar Dr. K Chang and Junior Dr G. Hudson of the neurology team, who oversaw the treatment for Myasthenia Gravis throughout my stay at Palmerston North Hospital. I thank you all.

Preface

This is my story. It provides some insight into how MG affects a person, the reasons for hospital admissions, and details of treatment approaches. At the end of this work I have included a list of resources, both local and national, clinical hospital terminology and clinical terminology specific to Myasthenia Gravis.

I use metaphors, describing the diagnosis as 'the elephant in the room' and this life-threatening (myasthenic) crisis as an MG Dragon. To me a dragon is magnificent, tyrannical, and deadly. One has to learn all about the dragon and how to ride it, to tame it. MG can be mild, moderate and manageable, or it can be debilitating and extremely deadly. Understanding the disease is key to managing it.

Those who have MG are affectionately known worldwide as 'snowflakes'. Each person has the core symptoms of the disease but each person's presentation and symptoms vary. The disease can be triggered by extremes in temperature, stress, and certain foods, but you may not know what the trigger is until after it has happened.

Every snowflake is intricate and beautiful, but no two snowflakes are the same.

In this book, there are a few other things I talk about in order to describe the whole experience of this illness. I didn't want it to be just a linear account of one thing: there were so many other processes that happened for me – psychological, spiritual, cognitive and emotional.

Finally, I wanted to put my story into a global context, to raise awareness that societal attitudes, governments, and even political change can affect the quality of life of the MG sufferer. It is a disease suffered alone, but whether the sufferer survives, gets to live a normal life, just exists, or dies, depends on the attitude, knowledge and actions of the society they live in. It is all of this that I want to share, to raise awareness, educate, enlighten and hope that my humble story will help to make change in the attitude towards, and treatment of, Myasthenia Gravis.

♥

Introduction

The 'elephant in the room' is the diagnosis. You find out what you have, but you have no idea what it is, how you come to have it, how it will affect you, or what questions to ask. It's a wait and see game. The 'elephant' is very much in your life, but you are too afraid to ask about it, and when you do, the answers are so left of field, that you realise it may be better not to know. Then, when eventually you do know more, the disease itself is so variable that you have to go through its many different phases to fully understand what it is – and how it is going to affect your life.

Before our children were born, our favourite thing was to go trekking. Sometimes my husband and I used to walk around the hills and walkways of the northland coast. It was always a great adventure going to the beach, and we loved to swim. Often he would go diving while I stayed 'sunning' myself on the shore. I had dedicated my married life to bringing up my children and taking care of my family. My husband worked while I was a stay-at-home mum. When the children started kohanga reo, I started voluntary work writing for a local newsletter for the Community House, and I stayed involved in the community for some years doing voluntary work.

Later, when our children got older, I kept fit by going to the gym. My husband was a coach for the local rugby league team, and sometimes he would take me through their training moves as well. I don't think I did so well with that, but the point is I liked to keep fit and physically healthy. I used to walk the children to school and pick them up from school. Walking has always been a favourite activity for me.

As time went on I returned as an extramural student to university. I gained qualifications from both Auckland and Massey Universities and did other training as well. I started to work in Human Services and in 2008 set up my own counseling consultancy. Life was getting on a roll as far as my career prospects were concerned, and it was an exciting time.

In late 2011, I was diagnosed with a rare autoimmune disease known as Ocular Myasthenia Gravis. This means grave muscle weakness of the face, eyes and jaw. I will refer to it as Myasthenia Gravis or MG from now on. Currently, the statistics in New Zealand for those affected with MG are ten in every 100,000 people. With our population of 4,602,802 that equates to approximately 460 people with some form of MG in this country. Having said that the number of diagnosed people registered with organisations like, NZ Myasthenia Gravis and Muscular Dystrophy Association, is far below that projection. The life-threatening 'Dragon crisis' I describe in this book hospitalised me for months. I have had crises before, but nothing like this one. I was to find that these Dragon crises are rare, a fact that poses challenges to treatment.

Now I know that in my case (as with 85% of diagnosed people) the disease has progressed to more of a generalised (whole body) status. This means that all skeletal muscles can be affected, either all at once or as muscle groups. The bulbar (mouth, face, throat, swallowing) and respiratory muscles (diaspora) are also affected, and that is where the life-threatening risk comes in; that is where the Dragon is most powerful.

There is a lot of literature out there on MG, but the number of people throughout New Zealand who actually present to hospital in a Dragon crisis is very small. Having said that, there are people who will present with differing levels of the disease, some of whom require neurology input and up to two weeks stay in hospital.

I found that when a condition is rare or uncommon, like Myasthenia Gravis, so too are the number of people knowledgeable in treatments of it. Any medical professional not familiar with MG who is 'lucky' enough to come across a person with this disease, will need to be prepared to research and understand it before treating. Consultation and collaboration with other medical professionals is important for tackling this potentially life-threatening disease. If a person presents to the Emergency Department (ED) in a Dragon crisis, their life is literally in the hands of the medical professionals.

There are two types of crisis that a person with Myasthenia Gravis will present with. Usually it is the lesser, ocular episode which affects the eyes (diplopia and ptosis), jaw, chewing, and speech (aphasia). This is not life-threatening but it can be disabling, preventing the person from driving, working and functioning normally. It requires neurology input; it doesn't just go away, and in fact it may worsen.

Another situation that can arise (reported by many sufferers of MG), is that they can be turned away from ED due to lack of knowledge by ED doctors. Sometimes the symptoms may be mistaken as psychosomatic or psychological and the person may be advised to simply make an appointment with their GP. Being turned away from the ED can be dangerous. Symptoms are just the tip of the iceberg and they worsen, not improve, over time.

The number of times the health system encounters a person in a life-threatening or Dragon crisis in New Zealand is very small, which is why patients with rare disorders such as Myasthenia Gravis have to be vigilant about their own health care. In an ideal world the health system would be very familiar with MG, its different presentations and corresponding treatments, just as it is with Diabetes, Rheumatoid Arthritis, and even Multiple Sclerosis (all autoimmune diseases), but the reality is that not many health workers know the different presentations of MG. As patients, I think it is our responsibility to describe as accurately as possible the symptoms we are experiencing. We also have to remember this is a two-way relationship and it's important to work alongside medical professionals to fight this disease. We can't expect medical staff to know about every rare medical condition that exists. I have found that the hospital encourages partnership between the patient and medical staff – it's a reciprocal, two way arrangement and the doctors are more open to patient input these days.

Other than actually interfacing with the health system in our everyday lives, appropriate self-care – managing physical exertion, diet, tasks and stressors – is important while we live with this disease. All of these aspects should be managed with the help of your consultants and neurologists. Myasthenia Gravis can vary in its initial presentation, and because of this, the medical professionals providing care and treatments need the information and resources to 'fight' the disease.

MG was once a terminal illness. Now there are a range of treatments available; the key is knowing how to apply them. Nowadays your neurologist will have that knowledge. There are quite a lot of resources on specialist medical websites, and specialist centres in Australia, USA and Great Britain that treat patients with Myasthenia Gravis. Now it is possible for both doctors and patients to research far and wide.

In Palmerston North Hospital, the team of neurologists are becoming familiar with the different aspects of the disease as there are about eleven people in the Manawatu Horowhenua/Tararua region with varying types of MG; we probably know each other, or go to the same support group. All of us have presented to the hospital at one time or another. Since last year when I was a patient at the hospital (April to September 2016), the hospital staff have been able to familiarise themselves with the complexities of this disease. The main medical units involved in my care were Neurology, Intensive Care Unit and Rehabilitation Star Ward 2. A multi-disciplinary approach to my treatment was taken and ultimately it was successful. I was discharged to my home and walked out of the hospital without aids or assistance on the 9th September 2016.

♥

Part 1

THE MG DRAGON
Myasthenia Gravis and life-threatening crisis

'To me a dragon is magnificent, tyrannical, and deadly. One has got to learn all about the dragon and how to ride it, to tame it.'

Chapter 1

The MG Dragon settles outside my door

In Oct 2011, I developed symptoms known as diplopia and ptosis and facial muscle weakness. The symptoms were extremely unusual, and of sudden onset. I had never experienced anything like it before. This was not in itself life-threatening or in the forefront of my thoughts, because I was unfamiliar with the symptoms and what they might mean. As time went on, when I couldn't see properly, it became a concern. The constant double vision interfered with everyday activities and commitments. My eyes were actually out of alignment, which I found out later was due to the ocular muscles weakening, impeding their usual function. I visited my GP and her assessment was that it was neurological, but not a stroke or Bell's palsy. At this early presentation and examination, she was unable to give a name to my condition, but suspected that something serious was going on. Little did I know that the MG Dragon had just settled outside my door.

My doctor put through urgent referrals to the

hospital and advised me to go to the Emergency Department (ED), if the condition worsened. The referrals took a very long time to be processed through the hospital system, and my symptoms did not abate at all.

That year, 2011, was a difficult one for our whānau. A culmination of many challenges had already been faced and it was also to be the last year we had our mother with us. As a whānau we supported and cared for our mother and each other during this time.

♥

Chapter 2

Visits to the Emergency Department of the Hospital

Late in 2011, I had to present to the Emergency Department of the hospital – not something I had ever had to do in the past. My symptoms had indeed worsened: my speech and chewing were affected and I was becoming very fatigued. I now know that these symptoms are serious indicators of an Ocular Myasthenia episode. The fatigue I felt was unfamiliar; my body felt heavy as well as tired.

These are the visible symptoms, indicators of what is happening in the body, and are a matter of serious concern. The disease itself goes a lot deeper, affecting the immune system and antibody production, which compromises the neuromuscular junction of the voluntary/skeletal muscles.

At this first ED presentation, the staff weren't sure what was wrong with me, and for a while I was kept in the rest area of ED. I did tell them I needed to be admitted as I could feel myself getting worse but, as I said, the ED doctors weren't familiar with MG.

Eventually I was put into the Medical Assessment and Planning Unit (MAPU) overnight. By the next day I was moved to a general ward, number 26.

The first appointment I had with the neurologist, Dr Carigas, was in the ward. As Palmerston North Hospital is a teaching hospital, he came with his students and examined me – my eyes, arms and legs. I had blood tests which he sent away to Europe to determine the diagnosis. He pondered whether it could be Guillain-Barre or Fischer syndrome, both autoimmune disorders, but it was neither.

The results returned from Europe a month later, confirming the diagnosis: Ocular Myasthenia Gravis. None of the other blood tests or nerve tests furnished many results; it was the antibody blood test that we had to wait for, and which gave up a result. The name of this disease was like a foreign language to me. It was good that I had a diagnosis because then I knew what I had to do, and what treatments to investigate, but not so good that somehow, out of thousands of people, I now had this disease which was in the 'rare' or 'uncommon' category.

Following the diagnosis, I was prescribed Mestinon (Pyridostigmine) by the neurologist, the usual treatment for Ocular MG, and my symptoms went away. I did quite well on that medication for a while.

As with most things, I had to adapt to a minor

change in lifestyle to 'accommodate' the demands of this disease. One of the main challenges was to come to terms with having the disease, and its implications. Even the term 'disease', which is what this is, can impact on a person's self-esteem and image. Outside the confines and safety of a hospital there is a certain amount of stigma due to misunderstandings attached to the term 'disease'. I have since found out that MG is neither hereditary nor contagious.

I've had a few trips to the ED (in 2013, 2014, 2015) with what I thought were crises. In hindsight they were minor episodes, not affecting my respiratory system much, but requiring an increase and change in medication, and sometimes IVIG treatment (the immunoglobulin Intragam P) five days in a row. This is an infusion that takes about four hours to complete. It has to be carefully measured and calibrated to the weight of the patient to minimise side effects; usually I have more benefits from this infusion than any adverse side effects. I was also started on the immunosuppressant Azathioprine. It had become necessary to control my immune system which now produced antibodies that worked *against* the neuromuscular junctions of my voluntary muscle groups instead of with them.

After a stay in hospital of about 5-10 days each time, I then went home to adapt to the new regime. Diplopia, ptosis and facial muscle weakness, voice absence or change were the main symptoms that were present with every episode. These symptoms are known as an Ocular MG crisis. This disease can start and remain with just the ocular symptoms, or it can also exacerbate and become generalised, affecting the whole body.

I took the immunosuppressant Azathioprine twice a day as part of my medication regime.
However, after two years of taking this medication, I developed an allergy to it. According to a pharmacist I spoke to, one can develop an allergy to Azathioprine even after long term use. This does not happen to many people, but it can happen. My ankles swelled up and I got a rash all over my arms. I took an antihistamine and that helped for a while, but with an allergy to medication, it is best to discuss it with your doctor and change or stop the
Medication − which is what I eventually did. Azathioprine does suit a lot of people, and it works well for many, so I was kind of unlucky that I had to give it up. I then went on to mycophenolate (Cellcept) − this is another immunosuppressant used to treat Myasthenia Gravis.

Research literature and commentary I've read on Myasthenia Gravis shows that it is not considered a progressive disease like Multiple Sclerosis, or Muscular Dystrophy. However, from talking to others with the condition and having MG myself, I've found that Ocular (facial) MG can advance to Generalised (whole body) MG. Other complications can worsen the situation, such as having a thymoma, and undergoing lengthy treatments or anaesthetics. Also, muscle weakness can take longer to resolve with each crisis, sometimes rendering muscles weaker in the long term. In some cases patients have to use mobility aids (especially for long trips) such as walking sticks, walkers or electric wheelchairs.

One small glimmer of light is that in many situations, MG is no longer terminal and can be controlled through medication and treatment. When the disease is manageable, people can and do get on with their lives. In some cases people have been known to go into remission.

♥

Chapter 3

Complications with Myasthenia Gravis: the Dragon returns, tyrannical and deadly

What makes MG even more complex to diagnose and treat is comorbid health conditions affecting the heart and lungs, as well as cancers and their treatments. Many of us don't think about how these can actually exacerbate the underlying condition of MG. But it can, and in my case it did. It's important to be aware of this, and to be as vigilant as you can about your own care by staying informed and communicating as much as you can. There may be times during your hospitalisation when you won't be able to communicate your needs. This is where whānau, family, friends or carers can advocate for you.

Invasive procedures like operations, anaesthetic, x-rays, CT scans, radiation therapy, and even a bout of pneumonia can aggravate any other underlying condition. In the last week of October 2015, I had to make an urgent dash to the ED of the local hospital. Although it was hard to imagine that something else apart from MG was wrong with me, it was also hard to think otherwise. I had a pain right in the centre of my chest, a type of sharp pressure – another unusual feeling that I had never experienced before. I thought, "Oh, no, is this a heart attack?"After some time in the ED, talking to doctors, having x-rays, and finally a CT scan, it was revealed that I had a thymoma in my chest behind my heart and lungs.

A thymoma is a tumour of the thymus gland, and is a common occurrence in people with MG. Standard practice is to remove the tumour when it is found. By the time the thymus in an adult is enlarged, it could be malignant and has to be removed immediately.

The thymus sits behind the sternum, below the thyroid gland, and carries out a critical function. It is a gland that builds the immune system from birth. Usually it is absorbed into the body during adolescence, but in some people it remains and becomes active, producing antibodies that act against the neuromuscular junction between nerve endings and muscles.

Obviously, I still had my thymus gland at the age of fifty-five, and by 2015 I was fifty-nine. Over this time my thymus gland had developed into a stage 2 malignant thymoma. When the thymoma was discovered my neurologist contacted the cardiothoracic unit at Wellington Hospital. The only option was a thymectomy, a resection of the thymoma, as soon as possible. It is usual procedure for a neurologist to refer an MG patient to the cardiothoracic unit and we attended a meeting with the cardiothoracic surgeon, Sean Galvin at Wellington Hospital. He made no attempt to minimise what I needed to understand and do. After this consultation, I had a further battery of tests of my heart, lungs and blood. I was booked in for surgery on the following Wednesday, 4th November 2015. He processed my referral rapidly and for that I am grateful.

My surgery was delayed and then deferred to the next day. On Thursday morning 5th November, I was wheeled in to the operating theatre. I really didn't know what was to come – open chest surgery was all new to me, but I knew it had to be done. It was definitely too late to throw my hands up in the air and run like the wind in the opposite direction.

The operation involved a cut through my chest wall and sternum (a sternotomy) as if for open heart surgery. The surgeon cut around the capsule of the thymoma, resecting it from the top of my heart and left lung where it was attached, and finishing with an artificial graft of my innominate vein. This is a brief explanation to describe a rather complex and lengthy operation of about five hours. The main thing I want to share is that the thymoma was removed, the 'capsule' it was in appeared intact and the surgeons said they 'got everything', so there was some consolation from what was quite an ordeal.

For many people with Myasthenia Gravis, a thymectomy is not necessarily long and complex. It depends on *when* it is found, whether it is benign or malignant, and the most appropriate way to remove it to ensure that all affected tissue is removed. There are different approaches to the surgery for different reasons.

♥

Chapter 4

Snowflake vs the dragon

At this point in my writing I have to sit and ponder how I have got this far. I never knew at that time, in 2015, what was going on within my body. In hindsight I was aware of my dwindling energy but thought it was residual MG from previous flare-ups, or a pulled muscle. One thing I'm glad about though, is that when I felt another unusual pain in my chest, I listened to my body: it gave me an alarm and I acted on it. I guess that is something we really have to take seriously – listening to our bodies. There is always a reason for pain.

I couldn't feel this onset of Myasthenia Gravis straight away; maybe it was too early in the piece. When I think back it seemed to be a development over time, from discovery of the thymoma (malignant) to the thymectomy, to another stint in Palmerston North Hospital in December 2015, to late March 2016 – this time with pneumonia after open chest surgery.

The 'Dragon' I feared was growing, intertwining itself around my organs, and coursing through my body. A Dragon massive in size, all powerful, rearing its head back, roaring and breathing fire. It was here, with me, in my head, a feeling in my body, ready to take away my very breath, and no one else could hear or see it. I had to face this Dragon alone. We all have a 'Dragon', and when it makes itself known to you, you have to learn how to fight it and tame it, because it's you or it. In March of 2016, my Dragon had just awoken. I knew I was entering a battle – I needed to pick my weapons well and fight back.

Even though my older sister and younger brother had other commitments, they gave up their time to be with me, coming down and attending my appointments so I didn't have to face the news alone. My sister stayed with me throughout the operation and hospital recovery, and afterwards looked after me at home. We pooled our resources, we worked together, and that's how I got through.

After the thymectomy, I was told by many well-meaning doctors, "Six weeks and you will be healed up and feeling a lot better." But it turned out that six weeks was quite naïvely optimistic of me (and them). Realistically it takes much longer, more like six months before all is 'good'. I was fifty-nine years old, a little bit fit from walking the big blocks at home, and a little bit fat from eating to replace the energy I'd just expended with all that walking … but it could have been much worse.

Within that space of six weeks − 3 months, I thought life as I knew it could have a chance to go back to normal, but I had other small routine procedures to do at the hospital. I'm aware now that every new invasive procedure on my body could easily have aggravated the MG, but at this time I wasn't suffering from any obvious symptoms of the disease, apart from a little fatigue.

Just around the corner, the biggest hurdle was the oncoming radiation therapy which was due to start in February 2016. This was to treat anything left from the thymoma, and was a critical part of the treatment.

I was ambivalent about my recovery needs. I think people do this all the time − leave ourselves out of the 'big picture'. Perhaps it's denial. I was busy thinking about work, income, maintaining normality, and not changing my routine to allow myself healing time outside of the six weeks. A big part of having a disease like Myasthenia Gravis is that it involves lifestyle changes, starting from the first flare-ups. In my case my stubbornness made me carry on, and now I know that that was not a good move. Rest is the best thing to do. Coming to terms with a disease like MG at an emotional level as well as an intellectual level was, and still is, hard to do. MG is a bit of a Pandora's Box − you never know what is going to come out next.

♥

Chapter 5

The Precipice

To me, at this point, my illness was like being on the edge of a precipice, looking down and not knowing if I would ever find a way out. January 28th 2016 was my three-hour planning session at the Radiotherapy Department of the hospital. During this time measurements were taken of where the thymoma had been, including the organs it was attached to. X-rays and CT scans were necessary to get as accurate a measurement and as much visual information as possible. Minimising the harm caused by the radiation to surrounding tissue and organs is critical. Several little dots are tattooed into the skin to provide a permanent mapping cue. This is normal procedure in preparation for radiation therapy.

On February 22[nd,] 2016 I had the first of my twenty-minute radiation therapy appointments. They were now to be at the end of every day, at around 3.30 pm, right through to April 1st 2016. I planned work around my treatments, because I had no idea of the side effects and how they would affect me. I would go home at the end of the day and rest up, or sometimes I would visit my cousin and stay in town. It worked for a while, and having talked to others, I found that they also continued to work (especially if they were self-employed), so I didn't think I was wrong in my decision to keep working. Having said that, if I'd had a more physical job, I would *not* have been able to continue working. It's about knowing your own limitations and what you can actually cope with.

Others who were undergoing radiation therapy at the same time as I was had to take leave from work, but most were older than me and if they were close to retirement, they were now planning to retire early. The noticeable difference between myself and others was that, as time went on, none of the people I spoke to felt the fatigue as much as I did. My fatigue seemed to progress and worsen with each week.

The treatment was charted for six weeks, but by the time I was into my fourth week I was really feeling fatigued. I developed diplopia (double vision) in my left eye – the first symptom of an MG onset. Later, other ocular symptoms such as jaw weakness and ptosis (drooping eyelid) set in. Thinking back on it now, I realise that my body had undergone a barrage of invasive treatments and procedures, but at the time I didn't make the connection that these symptoms were the beginning of an MG crisis of the most serious kind.

It was just a matter of time after that day. I

was worried that I had these symptoms and still two weeks of radiation therapy to go. I was between a rock and a hard place – I, and the radiation therapists, knew that the treatment was critical, and as far as I knew as a patient, there was no way around it. Radiation therapy is prescriptive and has to be delivered in doses over a set period of time to be effective. There seem to be no other options available. In hindsight (and for the benefit of other snowflakes) it is important to understand your condition, and that it can be aggravated by other procedures. Be aware of all potential risks.

My radiation therapy was completed on the 1st April 2016, and I was so relieved. It was critical that I completed this treatment, and I did. On that same day, I was quite weak and had to go again to the Emergency Department of the hospital, my friends in tow, and all of us with worried frowns. I think I may have been sent back home that time. However, on the 4th April I returned to the hospital and saw my neurology nurse, Rosie, who sat me down and asked me how I was. I said I was not that well and a bit short of breath. She then asked, "How long does it take for your breathing to deteriorate?" I told her it could be quick, and she immediately said, "I'm taking you to the ED myself." This she did, and made sure I got in straight away. That was lucky, because after that I deteriorated rapidly into an MG Dragon crisis. I had never experienced this before; I was in complete

42

collapse.

So here I was again in ED (April 2016) needing to be admitted due to another MG crisis. I was given respiratory testing (spirometry) by the ED doctors and my readings were lower than they should have been, but not startlingly low. I was also tested for muscle weakness in my eyes and arms, and for stamina – all were of interest. After the tests in ED, I was admitted and sent to MAPU, a triage unit. I was there for one night, then sent on to the ICU. On April the 7th I was put on nasal airflow tubes (Airvo) to keep my lungs inflated and oxygenated, then sent back to the Coronary Care Unit (CCU) on the 8th April. Two days later I was back in ICU. My brain seemed to be aware of what was going on, but my body had collapsed. I could no longer move any of my muscles.

Trying to breathe and sleep with the Airvo was impossible as the tubes blow full-on and non-stop right up your nose. I was focused on breathing but couldn't coordinate my ins and outs with the non-stop 'blast' of the Airvo. However, I kept up a good fight for as long as I could. My oxygen saturation readings were dropping down to the 70s; previously the normal range for me was 90 to 100%. CCU staff monitored this for a while, and noted that at night my oxygen readings would drop down so low they thought this was a risk and contacted ICU. At midnight on the third day (10th April) a number of nurses came to the unit dressed up in white gowns and masks and transferred me to the ICU.

The intensive care unit is a comparatively small ward with about eight bed spaces, but usually only six are occupied at any one time. Each patient is monitored and worked with according to their needs, so you are not left alone for long. Most patients who come to ICU can't perform the most basic bodily functions like eating, breathing, toileting and moving. Most of my previously taken-for-granted bodily functions were now being done by machines. I needed help with everything.

At this time in my writing, and with the benefit of hindsight, I can say that I have learnt much from this experience. For those with chronic illness who may go through this kind of trauma, I want to say, "Don't stick your head in the sand and don't take too long to act. Ask for help. People like to help where they can. No man is an island, so if you have a partner/spouse or children able to look after you – then good. If you don't, reach out to friends and whānau for help, because your healing and your resilience will be strengthened when someone is there to help and care for you."

If you are able, or if you have a family member or friend who can advocate for you, ask about community support such as home help, personal care assistance, social workers, and

Counselling. You can do this either through your doctor or from within the hospital.

It is really hard to get through such an illness alone. We all have to make that decision, to ask for help, when we get seriously ill.

♥

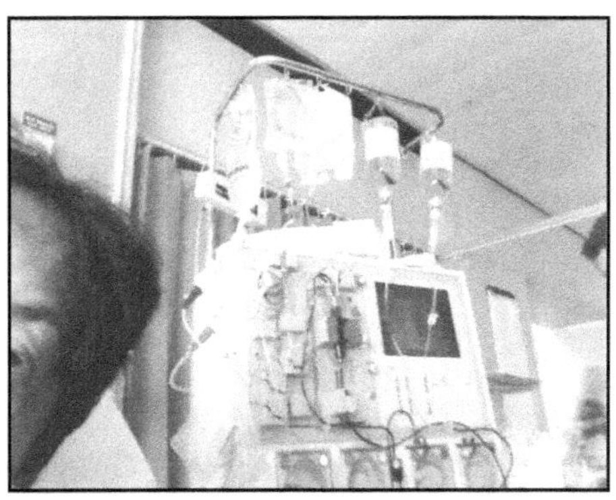

April 2016.
Coronary Care Unit, Palmerston North Hospital.

Plasmapheresis treatment crisis intervention after emergency admittance to hospital.

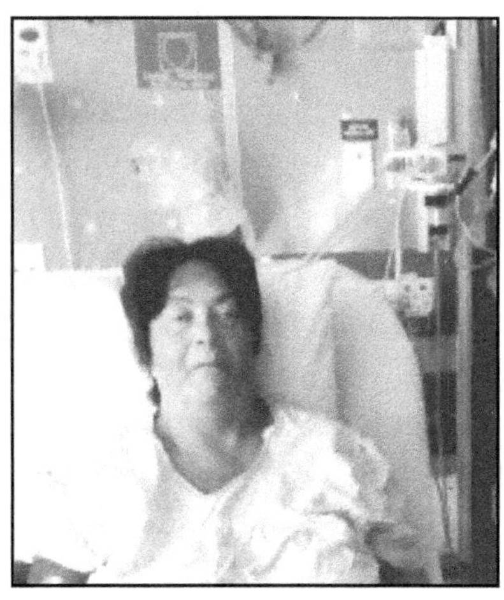

Chapter 6

Neurology Team

Dr Carigas, the consultant for neurology, working in parallel with the ICU team, started to work out a possible treatment plan. He looked at everything: the events that led up to my ED admittance and any previous procedures I had had done. There had to be a reason for this episode of MG and why it was so severe. Dr Carigas admitted that he had not encountered a crisis of this magnitude before. I'm so glad that he could take on the challenge of wading through the treatments to find one that was going to work for me.

Visiting me in ICU, he checked my charts and explained that they would do everything they could to get this MG Dragon under control. He admitted that it was a serious crisis and it could take a while. This was a precipice moment for me and his assurance meant everything.

Dr Carigas and his other team members starting talking to ICU consultant Dr Daniel Nistor, and a collaborative approach between the two teams was taken. The two front line treatments that are the most effective in treating MG are the immunoglobulin IVIg Privigen, and Plasmapheresis. These treatments tend to wash out all the antibodies from the blood, and I was able to have both. It was an aggressive approach, but it can be an aggressive disease, so the first line weapons were chosen for the first attack. Unfortunately, due to the type of crisis I was undergoing, its pre-emptive causes and other factors, the treatment did not work, and I deteriorated. In the team's experience this had hardly ever happened – until now. It was back to the drawing board.

While other specialist teams treated me in ICU, it was the neurology team who were responsible for treating the Myasthenia Gravis; mine was one of the most complex presentations of the disease they had ever had to grapple with. To me, the MG Dragon was growing more powerful every day.

The team monitored me fortnightly. Doctors Iniesto and Maata Rodriguez visited when they could and explained what they were doing, and monitored me whenever there was a change. Dr Carigas charted another approach to using the IVIg Privigen infusion and altered or increased my medications. They were calm and mindful in the middle of this crisis but also concerned as even though there was progress, it was miniscule. In the early stages it was almost unnoticeable. Dr Carigas and his team planned on another consistent and long term approach to my treatment which wouldn't set me back. It involved weekly immunoglobulin infusions on a Friday, an increase in immunosuppressants and Prednisone, and a continuation of Mestinon. The neurology team have their own unit and also visit patients in the wards. While I was being treated for respiratory failure in ICU, they were putting their treatment plan together.

The respiratory failure I had was typical of a severe Myasthenic Crisis: my breathing muscles weren't able to move, so I couldn't breathe in or out. This was not a result of the more commonly known causes of respiratory failure such as COPD, severe asthma, pneumonia or even lung damage. In my case it was simply that the nerves responsible for muscle movement were not able to send their signals to the muscle ends. Treatment was a two-pronged approach – addressing the muscle weakness (neurology team), and artificially keeping the lungs inflated and moving (ICU ventilator).

♥

Chapter 7

Battleground of choice: the Intensive Care Unit

During my 'stay' in the ICU unit, the head consultant responsible for me was Dr Daniel Nistor. The other important person that worked with him was the charge nurse, Sue Kirkman. It was to be a long stay, three months in total, and I got to know the nurses and unit well. I had to be catheterized to manage continence and my personal care was carried out by the nurses. They were always totally professional because they knew patients were not used to the huge changes they were going through.

On the 12th April I was started on the CPAP mask and I was on that for about ten days, intermittently with the Airvo. On the 25th, it looked as if I was coping quite well, when in reality, five days later I was struggling again − this seemed to be the nature of the beast I wrestled with. I continued to have further respiratory failure, to the point where any exertion, such as during a wash, caused me problems. I felt I couldn't lie flat as my lungs deflated more easily and were harder to 're-inflate'.

On the 30th April I had a cardiac arrest, and my heart stopped for thirty minutes.

This is what the registrar, Dr. Rau Fu, told me, as I was unconscious at the time. I cannot remember anything about stopping breathing, or the impact of CPR on my chest. I was lucky not to have broken ribs from the CPR as it went on for the full thirty minutes, and if it wasn't for the fitness of the registrar, well ... I hate to think. I had steel coils from my previous open-chest surgery holding my sternum together – and yes, it's still together! Other doctors and nurses were present during all of this, and maybe took turns with the CPR; I don't know any of the detail apart from what I was told by the registrar.

The intubation had helped by forcing air into my lungs, but now it was necessary to have something else to help me breathe, apart from the nasal flow (Airvo) tubes. This was to be a temporary measure, just one step down from a tracheostomy. While I was in ICU quite a few people had to be intubated because of respiratory weakness or failure. It took a bit of getting used to. Like the CPAP mask, I got used to it because it pushed oxygen into my lungs, which meant I didn't have to struggle to breathe in and out.

The CPAP mask was very tight, constricting, claustrophobic, and definitely not a good look, but there was no option. In fact it was actually a step up from the nasal flow tubes – at least you could relax and not have to struggle to breathe all the time. The mouthpiece of the intubation was also very restricting but it's something you have to put up with if you want to keep on living. Once I got used to it, I could relax and go back to sleep.

On the 2nd May, I had an episode of choking. My airway got blocked somehow during my sleep and I had to be assisted by the doctors. I had taken a sleeping pill, just to catch some much needed sleep, but this just dulled my senses and I don't think I could wake up enough to deal with the blockage.

Respiratory failure became more of a concern for the doctors and a tracheotomy was carried out on my throat, a trachie was inserted, and ventilator tubes were attached. As I was no longer being vented through oral intubation, a mixture of oxygen and room air was pumped into my lungs via the tracheotomy. Breathe in ... breathe out ... ahhhh. So began another two months on a ventilator which turned out to be both good and bad, as I will explain later.

At night when there was an emergency, there was noisy excitement as staff mobilised to accommodate new intakes. The vacant bed spaces had to be sterilised, changed around, and re-equipped. All new intakes were real life and death emergencies, babies, children, old and young people, people who had suffered massive strokes, pneumonia, attempted suicide, drug overdoses, car accident victims and so on. Victims of vehicle or other accidents are a harsh reality for ICU staff.

The staff worked tirelessly on every patient that came in. There was and is no easy task; the personal toll it must take on the staff is immeasurable. My instinct tells me that although at times it's gutting, heart-wrenching stuff, when a life is saved, it's all worth it. Going home at the end of the day doesn't necessarily mean one stops thinking about work, but it's a time to rest and reflect. Then another day rolls on, and the shift changes hands, and a new lot of bright shiny faces say, "Good morning."

Like most workers in the medical, care and helping professions they are brave hearts and I acknowledge them all.

♥

Chapter 8

An Epiphany

When I reflect on that week in early May, especially after my heart stopped and I underwent CPR, I remember spending some time in a void, in a world of grey shadows – and then there was a flicker of light from the room and the voice of the person performing CPR yelling, *"Come on, come on!"* I felt as if I was being sucked through a portal, back into the ward, with lights blazing and people surrounding the bed. I was told that it was Dr Rau Fu who continued CPR for thirty minutes to bring me back home. Even though I was unconscious, I was back. At that crucial time, a testing time, he saved my life. I don't think I can ever thank him enough, so I want to acknowledge here what he did for me and in turn, my whānau.

To face your mortality is a very 'edge of the cliff' experience – it's mind blowing, and to think that it happened to *me*, hits home. My mind went over and over the whole scenario. Things could have turned out very differently, and my world as I know it would be empty, everything in flux, and my children enduring more suffering. I just can't stand the thought of that – if I had *really* died I mean. Technically I did die, but luckily I came back, so I guess it's not my time yet. I think it's always a message though when something like that happens to a person, and you just thank your lucky stars you're still alive.

I guess those who would know more about what happened would be my siblings who I heard had come to the unit to be with me, as the ICU doctors were not sure that I would survive. I'm assuming the nurses started ringing them when I went into cardiac arrest. It seems to be protocol to let the families and whānau know how their loved one is, and when to come into the unit. This happened many times to others in the ICU whose prognosis was doubtful.

On the same night that I was intubated and put on the ventilator, I was given adrenalin to keep my heart pumping. When I woke up I was quite aware of being awake, but I had no memory of anything that had happened. I looked around and I could see my brothers, sister and sister in law leaning over the bed. There was muffled conversation, laughs and sniffles and I just looked at them not really knowing why they were there. Was it visiting hours already? And yet it was still dark. No, it wasn't visiting hours – my whānau had been called in.

I said, "Hey what are you guys doing here?" They said, "We've come to see you! What's going

<u>May 2016 ICU</u>

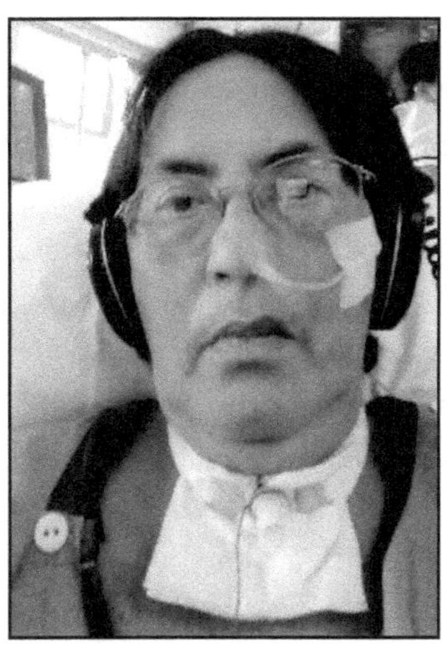

Listening to the TV.
"Trachie" in my throat
helps with breathing and
swallowing.

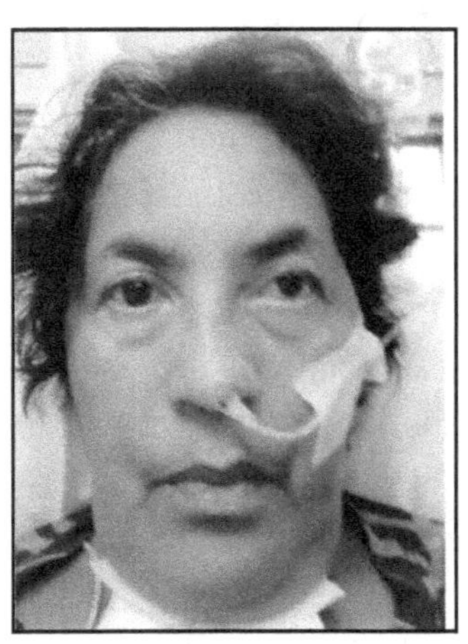

Nasogastric tube is in. I
received all
nutrition and medical through
this tube.

on?" I didn't realise at the time that my sister had boarded the midnight flight from Auckland to come down, and everyone had rushed from their houses in the middle of the night just to be by me. It was such a whirlwind of events, my head still spins when I think about it. My siblings, my whānau, are staunch to the end, never complaining or bringing it up, just getting on with their lives. They moved through the trauma of losing their youngest sister, a mother to their niece and nephew, to keeping her, and that's the best ending to this bit.

In my professional life I helped people deal with their own 'Dragons'. Now I had to reach down deep and pull some of those psychological skills to the fore. To keep things real, I had to find a way to stay in the present.

During visits I couldn't talk or show much expression, and it was quite hard for visitors
who wanted to comfort me with their words and conversation, including my children, and that saddened me. I did my best but I couldn't respond as I wanted to. To stay grounded I thought of my children and my whānau. All of the things I took for granted were now not available to me … apart from a drawing board and a felt tip whiteboard marker. Now that was a light bulb moment!

I conversed through words on the whiteboard.

Now at least I could answer people and they knew I was listening and interested. Of course I was:

their faces, their voices, their touch and karakia were the healing balms that fed my wairua, and that helped me be strong. That's why my visitors came, to give me that strength, and to let me know I would be OK. When there were emergencies, crises, usually I just lay there waiting for daylight. I was an ICU patient so I couldn't get out of there. I could barely turn onto my side and, like the other patients, I had to cope somehow. As you would expect in ICU, it is quite noisy with the constant beeping of medical machinery. In this hurly burly place of emergencies and crises, I would go into my own world and feed my imagination with thoughts, ideas and visions.

I think my ability to do this, to create my own illusions, kept my mind strong. Having that detachment gave me an excuse to just close my eyes and drift away, into a half sleep. I knew that it would be morning soon. During the day, as time went on, I managed to stay awake more and more. I started to interact more, I talked with the staff and joked around, listened to music and held people's hands, did my physio exercises, and met with the doctors every morning to map out my plan and progress. All of these things kept me focused on getting better.

My inner conversations though were sometimes very different to what I actually said or wrote down on the whiteboard. Sometimes it was a struggle that I couldn't or wouldn't articulate. A fear that lurked in the back of my mind was that I wouldn't make it, despite all the time that was spent on me, and the fact that I was now on a ventilator didn't bode well. As I erred on the negative, my feelings and my emotional state were a little vulnerable. I have to say when you are suffering such a loss of health, it's not *irreversible*, but it's daunting, like never seeing the top of the mountain. In this darkest time I hadn't seen either of my children, and I missed them very much. What I did have was their photos, so I focused on those, and knew I had to stay strong for them. Actually one of the strongest motivations to keep me on track was thinking about my children, from when they were babies, right up to now. Our ups and downs, our impossible times, our insurmountable odds and our little lights at the end of the proverbial tunnel. Funny what you think about. But hey, that's what family is all about, and that's the 'glue' that keeps us connected, through anything and everything.

♥

Chapter 9

Dieticians in ICU

Various interventions were happening simultaneously while I was in ICU, and the dieticians were involved regarding nutrition and feeding regimes. In March, my ability to chew food, and my appetite dissipated quite rapidly, by April I had lost almost fifteen kilos.

Further weakness of my bulbar (oesophageal/swallowing) muscles, meant the nasogastric tube was the only option to administer the nutrition and medication I desperately needed. My body was failing, and a decision had to be made as to how to keep it going while I continued on in ICU.

The nasogastric tube should be put in by a trained and experienced doctor as it can be painful and cause damage to your nasal passage if installed in the wrong way. Once I had experienced this (the latter), I made sure to ask for a doctor to do this procedure. They also used a nasal numbing spray to ease the sharpness of the tube going through my nasal and throat passages into my oesophagus.

Nasogastric (NG) feeding is one of the

specialist areas of dieticians, and is a more technical, scientific side to their role. Margaret was the dietician who worked in the ICU. Friendly and easy to talk to, she went about her work, keeping an eye on everything to do with the feeding regime. She charted a feed mix that was protein rich, to keep my muscles from starving and wasting. It was also high calorie so I had some energy. In normal circumstances 'energy' is something we take for granted. In ICU, you have none, you may be on bed rest for weeks. In order for patients to be able to transfer out of ICU to another ward, they have to start mobilising more than just turning over in bed! Lung and muscle function must be increased, as well as building and maintaining muscle strength. I learnt this after a while, and got to understand the whys and wherefores of my treatment.

The feed was monitored regularly by Margaret, due to the volume of liquid in the feed, the need to flush the NG tube and balance it all with the medications and fluid that I was having, either through the tube or IV. She also had to monitor the millilitres per hour/volume to ensure I was getting the exact level of nutrition required for a 24/7 feeding regime. That was how it was in ICU: no food at all, only liquid feed via the nasogastric feeding tube in my nose. Sounds scary, but it kept me alive, and there was no chance of weight gain!

From then on, when it came to food, taste, texture, anything, I learnt to eat with my eyes. I devoured images in magazines, on TV, and anything else I noticed about food. I guess that was my way of keeping in touch with reality. I wasn't going to just turn my mind off food.

Officially I now had Myasthenia Gravis Generalised. In 85% of cases, the disease can progress to a generalised state which affects the whole body. Unlike those with the *generalised* diagnosis though, MG weakness in my larger global muscles (legs, back) resolved faster than my ocular and bulbar muscles. I was able to mobilise with assistance way before I could eat and swallow. I still had ongoing diplopia, ptosis, and facial muscle weakness. Unlike other autoimmune disorders, in MG a life-threatening crisis begins when the respiratory muscles are hit. When that happens, you know you are in trouble.

The ventilator took over when my respiratory muscles weakened. I wasn't going to play Russian roulette with my odds; after all they weren't that great and I needed all the help I could get. I had read in all the MG literature that forced ventilation can happen when there is a serious MG crisis, so it wasn't totally unexpected − more like another part of the process in my treatment. Yes, in hindsight that is easy to say. As long as I kept the notion in my mind that I knew what to expect, I felt in control.

♥

Chapter 10

Physiotherapy in ICU.

This is where the energy is needed! There is no getting away from the fact that a ventilator and a nasogastric feeding tube are machines that are keeping you alive. You can't go anywhere until you are 'transitioned', which means detaching from the permanent fixed machine to a portable one. In my case it took a few people to help with everything that needed to be done for this to happen. The old saying 'Where there's a will there's a way' took on a new meaning for me! Each foray into physiotherapy was a combined effort by the physiotherapists, the nurses, and me. Sometimes I would be so exhausted by the end of a little walk around the unit, I would have to sleep for about two hours, and sometimes I fell asleep in the middle of an exercise.

It got better as the weeks went on, the nurses and physio's going with my flow, encouraging me, and clapping when I got back to the unit from doing the 'full circuit'. I didn't think I could do a lot of this stuff, but I did it, and that's the thing – you just do it. You have to have faith in yourself.

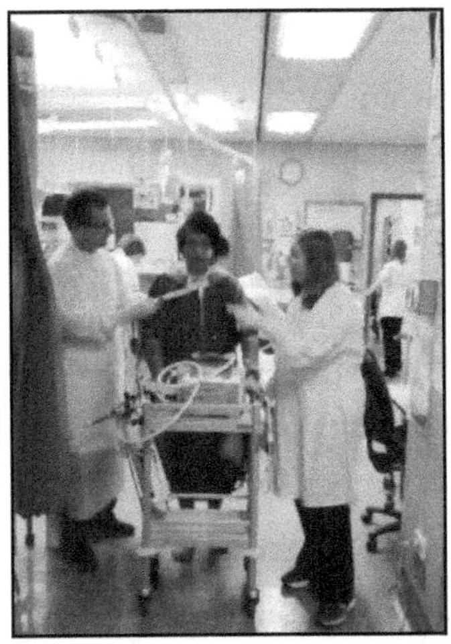

<u>May/June 2016</u>
<u>ICU</u>

Physiotherapy in the intensive care unit.

Malcolm - ICU Physiotherapist

Becky - ICU Nurse

Walking around the unit.

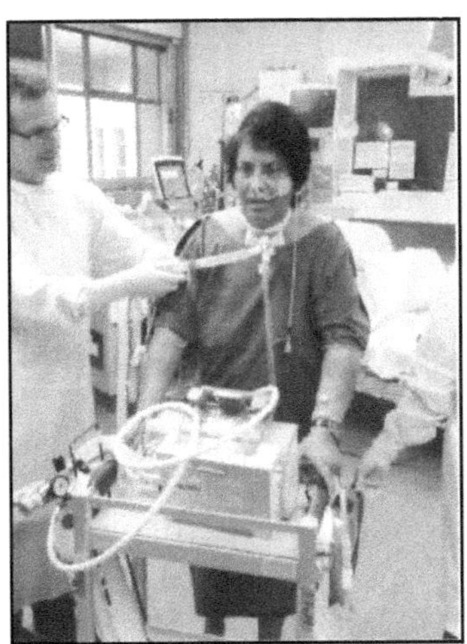

Malcolm helping me with walking exercises in ICU.

Malcolm was my physiotherapist in the ICU. His clever wit was his trademark and when things were a bit gloomy, he always kept the mood light. He took things in his stride; some days when I didn't or couldn't do physio it was never a problem, we just started again the next day. His consistent approach to my physio, albeit slow to start off with, helped me to strengthen my respiratory ability and ultimately get off the ventilator. This was my sole focus.

Disconnecting and reconnecting to life-giving machinery whenever I wanted to go somewhere may not sound like a big deal, but it was disheartening because I wondered what it would be like if I had to 'live' like this permanently. The doctor had talked about this possibility with me. It was not a *definite*, but it was an alternative should things not go as expected. Over time, disconnecting and reconnecting to this machinery became routine if I wanted to go anywhere, otherwise I simply didn't go. To keep my brain active, I observed a lot about the machines and learnt a little about how they worked, especially the nasogastric feeding regime, the ventilator and how it measured my breathing and lung capacity, and then the weaning process. From that point on I strengthened my resolve as well, and focused on recovery.

Another hurdle was the trachie which was inserted into my throat, through the cartilage and under the thyroid gland to sit above my vocal chords.

I couldn't talk and it was a challenge to manage. It interfered with the natural process of breathing through my nose and mouth, and I had to have a humidifier attached to maintain moisture in my airway. Usually the nose or the nasal passage naturally maintains the right humidity for the mouth, throat and breathing passage.

The trachie regularly needed to be suctioned via a plastic 'yankuer', and sometimes right in the actual trachie opening via a long tube. It interfered with my ability to swallow, up to a point. To those readers who are snowflakes (people who have MG), I persevered with it because I had to have another means to breathe, and later to prevent aspiration, *so I reiterate*, if you need a tracheostomy, it's because you absolutely do; it is never done unless it's necessary. Sometimes it is a temporary measure and not in for long.

Not being able to do much physically, locked away in my little world, right in the grip of an MG Dragon, I sometimes wondered about my future prospects, and if there even were any. These thoughts and feelings are normal. It's not a crime to have them; they are part of the process of clearing, so when you come through the haze, and you reach your 'clearing', then you can make changes. Hold on to good memories and to your strengths, and options will present themselves to you.

When I got visitors, I could always use my

whiteboard and whiteboard marker and I would write things down. Although it was a blessing to be able to write, it wasn't the same as the ebb and flow of conversation – but it was the next best thing.

♥

Chapter 11

Serendipitous moments

Whenever there was an opportunity to do something or go somewhere, I grasped it. The ICU nurses, if they weren't busy, would take me on walks around the hospital, down to the ATM machine, out to the 'Garden of Tranquillity'. They were awesome. Sometimes they painted my nails; I would regularly have a different colour of nail polish to show or surprise the visiting doctors with. It was fun, and certainly kept my spirits up.

Lyn, the education nurse from ICU, introduced new games to help me start focusing on other things and use my thinking skills. I don't think I was very good at them, but those were cool times I won't forget, and now (several months later) I am working my way through a huge crossword book. The charge nurse of the ICU, Sue Kirkman, arranged for visits with my disabled daughter. We would head off to the Whare Rapuora (Maori Health Unit) and they were wonderful − hosting the visit, playing music and making us a light morning tea.

68

Sue and Lorraine Searancke (Whare Rapuora) organised this for me and my daughter, and it was wonderful. I hadn't seen my girl for a while so it was a godsend to have her visit and be happy to see her mum. The ultimate for me was being able to *see* her – me being tied to all the machinery and not being able to talk to her hindered our usual way of communicating, but never mind, we had a little cup of tea and a bicky and we were good.

Sue and Lorraine also arranged for the ukulele group (the Kaumafias) from the whare to visit the ICU unit (this had never been done before) and later the rehabilitation unit, where everyone got to enjoy their fabulous music. I still have their mini-concerts on the video recorder in my phone. It's a record of our lighter, happier moments in the ward and the sheer kindness of people, especially Sue and the Whare Rapuora Kaumafias Ukulele club. They were awesome.

When there was no show of going anywhere else, I really enjoyed the impromptu trips out of the ward, just down to the front main entrance to the hospital. Sue was awesome, always thinking outside the square. It helped me, it really did, as my inner world got an airing, and I could see other people and buy something from the chemist and just breathe.

Those serendipitous moments helped me to build faith in my ability to survive, and although their results are intangible, they are also indisputable. For all that Sue had to do in terms of her own work as the charge nurse of the ICU, managing staff and intakes into the unit, she gave some thought to what I may need to boost my recovery. I don't think I will ever forget how thoughtful and kind she was.

Going for a walk with me was never straightforward. Usually Sue had to make sure everyone was available, and that there was enough staff on to accompany me, and also to staff the ICU. We made several trips to the hospital main foyer, complete with recliner chair (and much later the wheelchair), trolley, oxygen, portable suction, Dr Daniel (who always made himself available) and two nurses. It was a bit like a wagon train, but we did it and I loved it.

We would get outside and sit in the sun, people-watch, glance through the odd mag if we had one, chat and laugh about life. Once, I spent time with my visitors outside as they were coming in just as we had settled in a sunny spot. Those little silver linings were life-savers. The humour of the nurses was also something that lightened the mood of the ICU ward. They always found something to laugh about, or had lovely recipes to swap − a bit of home, and a bit of normality in their work world. I even bought some beautiful free-range eggs from one of the nurses − I wanted them for my whānau who had been visiting regularly, just as a treat for them. I would love to get some more of those for my own pantry one day.

♥

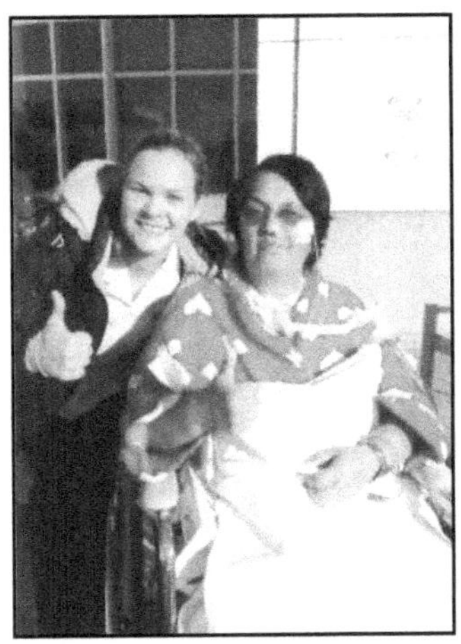

June 2016 ICU

ICU Nurse Fiona and I out and about at the hospital. I am attached to a mobile ventilator.

Visiting with my daughter at the Whare Rapuora. L-R Sue, (ICU Charge Nurse), Daniel (ICU consultant), Ashley (ICU Nurse)

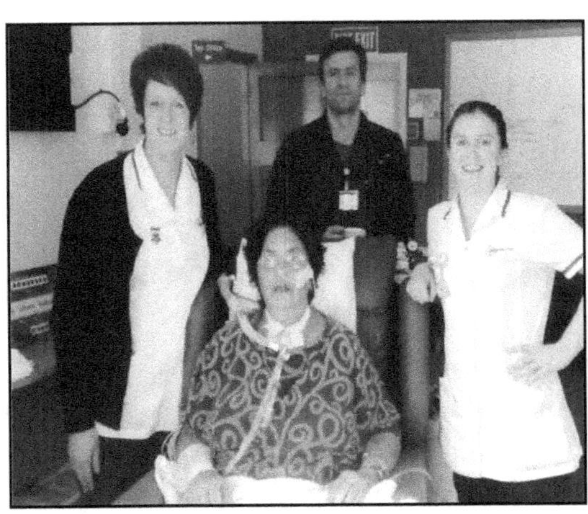

Chapter 12

Discharge from Intensive Care Unit, three months later.

Taming of the MG Dragon.

I was in ICU for April, May and June, almost a record! But by the end of June I was ready for discharge from ICU to another ward and then to the Rehabilitation Ward. Now the MG Dragon was diminishing, growing smaller, and I was progressing. Over the whole month of June, I was weaned off the ventilator under the supervision of Dr Daniel Nistor. He kept a vigilant eye on me during this time. There were moments of concern, but then it was just a process to go through. He encouraged me every day, always staying realistic, aware of the pitfalls should things go wrong, but I gathered from his concern that for him, it wasn't just about a patient and treatment, it was about a person who really needed things to go right.

It was the night times that were difficult: going into a deep sleep meant my oxygen uptake could drop to very low levels and the nurses would have to turn the ventilator up, which counteracted any weaning. Or I could stop breathing, or choke − so yes, there were concerns all the way through. All this was connected to MG and its effect on my bulbar and respiratory muscles. Having said that, I will never forget the dedication Daniel showed, not just to me but to all of his patients. He was awesome. Without the care and expertise of consultants like him, the outcome may have been very different.

Having had respiratory physiotherapy in the ICU, I had a little head start on improving my mobility and by June I was able to walk short distances around the unit, wash with help, and move on to my side. My breathing was much improved, and because of everyone's efforts I was able to be discharged from ICU. I was so happy about that, and so were the ICU staff.

One of the main goals of ICU staff is to be able to discharge patients towards rehabilitation, because it means the person is through the worst of their ordeal and on their way home. I think that for them, seeing a person move forward in their recovery is a highlight, and a reward for all their hard work. On the 28th June I was transferred to Ward 26, which was very busy and not equipped to help me properly with the tracheostomy, and nasogastric tube. I couldn't converse with anyone, and I was noisy, which didn't endear me to any of the other patients. I still needed a lot of help as well. Rehabilitation was my next main stay and it meant that I was finally 'on the mend'. I was transferred there on the 5th June.

♥

Part 2

Specialist Services within the Hospital (1)

Chapter 13

Rehabilitation Ward

The Rehabilitation Consultant that I came under was Dr. John Bourke; he was in charge of my treatment and progress. Regular Multi-Disciplinary Team (MDT) meetings were where information was discussed and decisions made about each patient. Dr Bourke had a good overview of my treatment while in rehab, as all medical notes were recorded by each nurse and therapist. From there he could assess where I was in my rehabilitation and the best time for discharge from the ward. Treatment plans had input from the whole team, encouraging a very comprehensive approach. He usually did his rounds accompanied by his registrar and junior doctors.

Judith was the charge nurse, Marie and Mary the assistant charge nurses – three very experienced and skilled managers who oversaw the nursing staff and activities on the rehabilitation ward. They were always approachable, friendly and professional, with staff and patients alike. At each shift, the nurses do their handover and come and say hi, and carry on with their duties. They are professional, skilled and specialists in rehabilitation, encouraging patients towards progress. Sometimes it's a fine balance between knowing when to encourage and when to step back. Each patient is different, as are their abilities. Some nurses were over-eager, pushing us to rehab quickly, while others understood completely what it took to rehabilitate. There was never any shortage of work to do. The nurses went about their business helping patients from early morning to bedtime, and sometimes during the night when patients were distressed, or not able to sleep. While specialist therapists worked with patients towards their rehabilitation, the 'engine room' of the ward was run by the vast number of nursing staff and care assistants who work in the background, solidly, 24/7.

Here I'd like to say a special thank you to Moa, the Specialist Clinical Nurse, who booked me my own room, with a TV. I was able to rest and rehabilitate and after a two-month stay it was a very good call! The Care Assistants, Jocelyn, Michelle and Eleanor, were so kind, helpful, and hardworking, doing all sorts of jobs around the ward as well as working alongside the nurses. They were always helpful to the patients. No job was too tough; they just got in and helped without complaint. I was one of those patients that had to be helped a lot, and it was humbling. This was the first time I had noticed just how much they do, so I know they are an asset to any ward and keep the 'engine room' of the rehab ward running smoothly.

♥

Chapter 14

Time for Rehabilitation

When I arrived at the rehabilitation ward, I still had difficulty doing things for myself. I needed assistance with just about everything. I guessed it was going to be a matter of building confidence, muscle strength and motivation, as well as an exercise regime. After all, I had had a few practice runs while in ICU. I still had the tracheostomy and nasogastric feeding tube in as a precaution. The bulbar muscles affected by MG were still to resolve in order for me to be able to eat, drink and swallow normally.

I continued on the feeding tube because there was a real risk of aspiration. The trachie now served as a protection for my windpipe; it had a small balloon attached at the bottom that blocked any food or drink from going into my lungs. Both of these attachments were cumbersome and alien, but there is a time when one has to just accept that 'it is what it is' and put up with the nuisance of being attached to machines. The difference for me was that I was like that for almost five months.

When I saw the Clinical Specialist nurse – Moa from Rehabilitation Star Ward 2, I was very happy to plan my goals with her, which included being free of both the trachie and the nasogastric tube. It was to be a straightforward course – *of course!* A pragmatic approach and why not? By now I was off the ventilator, which I have to say, was a great achievement for me. I was now free to move around a little more.

On August 2nd when I was transferred to Room 11 in Star Ward 2, I was swallowing my saliva more, and as the trachie had been in for a very long time (four months), it was finally removed. This was on the condition that I kept the NG tube in to cater for my nutrition and medical needs – no eating or drinking orally – and I had to keep up with the oromotor and facial exercises with the Speech Language Therapist, Marie Jardine. Having the trachie out helped me to get used to breathing through my nose and mouth again and did away with the extra attachments. My healing from the tracheostomy was gradual and took a few weeks, during which time everything slowly went back to normal. Having said that the tracheostomy does leave a scar on your throat that is visible, and there will also be scar tissue within the windpipe. This is normal. There may be infections and breathing complications further down the track, but they are usually treatable. It takes time, maybe even months for everything to go back to normal. The main thing is to look after yourself and keep faith in your ability to survive. And do what you can to never have it done ever again!

On the 19th August, well ensconced in my rehab room 11, the day had been a good one. I was off the nasogastric tube and, having had all my swallowing assessments and a video x-ray of my oesophagus, I was approved to have drinks and pureed food. Everything was so delicious! However, unexpectedly I had another setback: my swallowing and facial muscle weakness returned after a day of eating, drinking, swallowing and talking, an overload of activity on my oesophageal muscles. By the evening I was quite exhausted and stressed and swallowing was the last thing I should have done. My medication was missed that evening, and in the morning I was unable to function properly. My face and tongue were swollen; I couldn't speak or do anything. The doctors were called in and I was back to ICU.

The house doctors provided medical intervention for the muscle weakness and the consultant for ICU, Dr Nistor, helped to get my breathing right and settled into a regular pattern. I had to have the nasogastric tube refitted, and start again. I agreed readily, because this way medications could be re-administered which helped to de-escalate the muscle weakness, and the next day I was nearly back to normal. It certainly was a wake-up call − that sometimes gains should be gradual and monitored at each step. MG does not behave in a 'logical' way; symptoms can fluctuate on their way to resolving, especially at the tail end of a crisis.

What did I learn from this? Don't be in a hurry, and that applies to everyone involved in your care. It *is exciting* to witness progress, but being aware that MG symptoms can fluctuate is key.

♥

Chapter 15

Dietician in the Rehabilitation ward

The dietician to take over my care in the rehabilitation ward was Peter Heald, a young man of few words, who was diligent in his work. He made sure I had the right feeding regime in this ward. I needed something to provide me with energy for my rehabilitation activities, so the feed was set at 2000 calories a day. I had continued to lose weight so that level of calorie intake seemed appropriate. I'd also had the nasogastric tube for an unusually extended length of time, so Peter would make sure I had the right feeding lines available to the nurses, as these had to be changed and flushed regularly. My medications were still in liquid form and able to be 'injected' into the nasogastric tubing. Now I realise how helpful it was to have that tube. Yes, it was uncomfortable, and yes, it felt alien in my nose and throat, but it helped towards my recovery through nutrition and medication − then my two priority needs.

Peter would also make sure that I had enough

'bags' of feed in store as I started on a 24/7 regime, so each bag had to be replaced as soon as it was completed. If a bag was missed, (which could happen overnight) I would be very weak the following day, and would not be able to do much but sleep until my energy returned.

As time went on, and after input from the Speech and Language Therapists (SLTs), I was able to experiment with swallowing drinks and some foods. It wasn't always successful, but I continued to work at it with the SLTs and continued to have assessments of my swallowing muscles. Eventually they started to work again.

When this happened, and it was safe to try eating and drinking with the NG tube remaining in place, the feed was set down to 1800 calories, and then changed to twenty hours a day with a four-hour break, followed by eighteen hours a day with a six hour break. In this way I was weaned off the nasogastric tube, and now as I write this I can say I've been off it since the 31st August, so it's been six days without incident. It was good to talk to Peter today (6th September) and to see a relaxed smile on his face as we briefly summed up the whole process. I think we were both relieved to look back on the progress I had made. I was moving forward rather than facing the prospect of going home still dependant on feeding tubes.

♥

Chapter 16

Speech Language Therapy

Once again I discovered something new – that the skills of the Speech Language Therapists go beyond helping people to talk and form words. Their role in the hospital branches into a few areas: they assist patients who have had strokes, brain injury, head and neck cancers, and developmental delay, as well as autoimmune illnesses. They helped patients regain their ability to swallow and to speak. In my case, Myasthenia Gravis affects my bulbar, oesophageal, head, neck and ocular muscles. While in crisis, these muscles stopped working. With careful guidance from the Speech Language Therapist, Marie, I learnt oromotor, soft palate and safe swallowing, lip sealing and voice care exercises. Firstly, to prompt my swallowing muscles to start to behave as they normally would, and secondly, to get used to moving my mouth and tongue muscles, as I hadn't had to use them for a few months to eat, swallow or talk. My oromotor muscles had worked before, and like most people, I didn't notice what they did or how important they were until they stopped working! The exercises Marie was teaching me were to prompt them to start up again. I had FEES (Fibre optic Endoscopic Evaluation of Swallowing) assessments every two weeks to see how my swallowing muscles were progressing, and I was getting there. This involved a minute camera on the end of a tube, pushed up into the nasal cavity and down to the larynx and vocal folds. Jody, the senior of the two therapists, carried out the more technical side of the assessments.

I had seven FEES in total, and one Video fluoroscopic Swallowing Study (VFSS), which provided an x-ray of a side view of my oesophagus and showed how food travelled to my stomach. Both Jody and Marie attended the barium swallow. These kinds of assessments are carried out and interpreted by a radiology doctor.

My assessment showed that my swallowing had returned to normal, and the oesophageal motility of bolus to my stomach was not showing anything of concern. Everything was clear and normal. It also showed that my vocal folds, which had previously caused me stridor (a harsh vibrating noise when breathing) were now opening as they should. I knew at this time that Jody and Marie weren't taking this situation lightly; they wanted to make sure they were doing all they could to help me.

As a patient I would not have been aware of what could be done or the work involved, were it not for the methodical approach taken by both Jody and Marie.

The most important memory I have of this intervention is that it informed me that I could get help to swallow, eat and drink normally, and talk again – something I thought may not happen! And, I had an inside knowledge of what my oesophagus was doing! This may seem strange, but when you've been fed through a tube for nearly five months, eating and drinking normally, becomes uppermost in your thoughts.

To Jody and Marie, me regaining normal eating, drinking and swallowing were achievable goals, but it was going to take a while, and for my part, I had to trust that they were specialists in what they did. At the end of our hard work, my swallowing returned. I could eat and drink normally and the nasogastric tube was removed for the last time. I'm very grateful for the help given to me by Marie, especially as she visited me daily and put me through my exercises, and made sure I had homework over the weekend – all so that I would reach my goals.

On reflection, I know that to begin with I wondered about these strange exercises, and whether or not they would work. Now I know that they not only worked, but were critical for helping me get my normal life back.

♥

<u>June 2016</u>

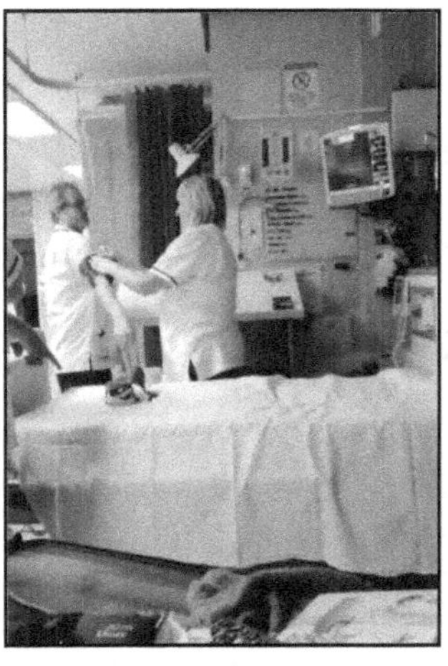

Lighter moments

"ICU but you do see me!!"

Pete and Andrea ICU nurses check the blood pressure equipment.

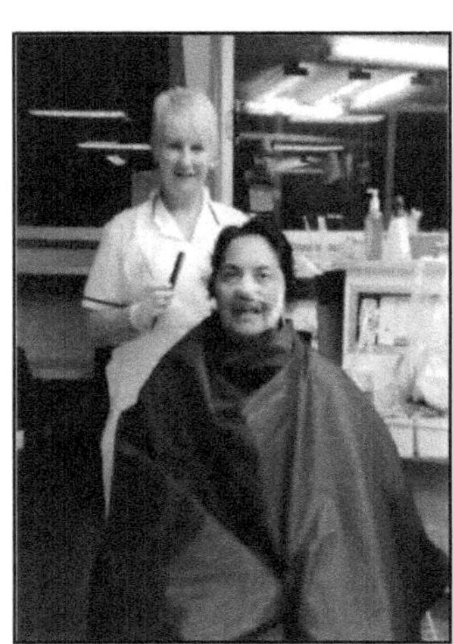

Having a hair cut with ICU Nurse Jane.

August 2016

Rehabilitation ward - STAR 2.

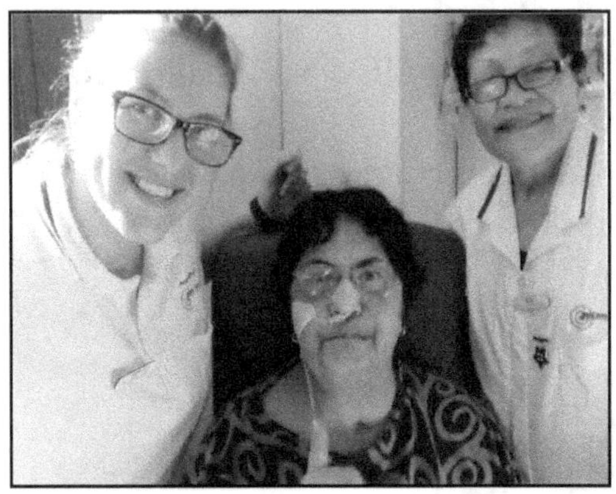

L-R Jaimee - Physiotherapist in Rehab. Ward and
Moa - Clinical Specialist Nurse.

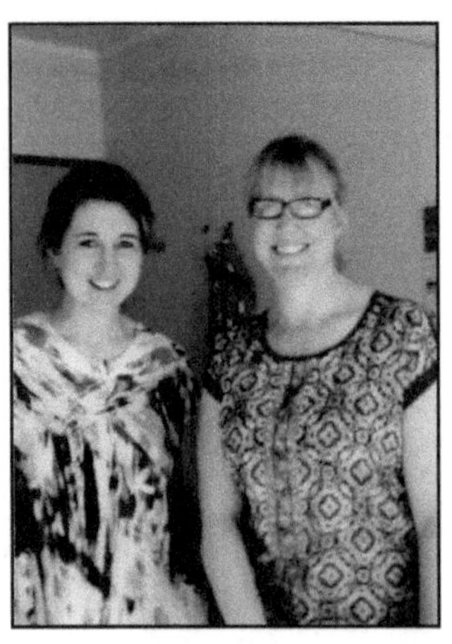

Speech language therapists
Marie and Jodi.

Chapter 17

Physiotherapy in the Rehabilitation Ward

My physiotherapist in rehabilitation was Jaimee. She brought young energy to our work. Although young in years and in the work itself, she put a good program together that suited where I was physically, and how I could progress. She also researched information on Myasthenia Gravis, which I thought was very good for me and anyone else with MG with whom she may work in the future. There was no room for feeling sorry for myself when it came to physio, I still had to do all of the exercises. However, when I just couldn't go to physio or do much, I would stay in my room and sleep.

When we began our work, I needed the wheelchair and the mobility walker, as I was quite weak and wobbly. After physio I was exhausted and would sleep for hours as my body started to meet the demands of the exercises. At that stage there weren't a lot of them – taking maybe fifteen minutes at the most. In the afternoon I continued with the Inspirometry Muscle Training (IMT) exercises to improve my respiratory strength. Jaimee would take me through these and sometimes we would play games like hangman, I spy, native animals and plants of New Zealand. It was fun.

After four weeks my 'global' or larger muscles started to move normally. The walker became my friend, and I got quite attached to it. It was a seat when I got tired, I could put my things in the basket and hide them, walk around the corridors of the unit, I could be pushed around on it, and I could go on little drives. But eventually I had to let it go, and even though it took nearly two months, I did let it go. Guess what? I'm OK. Looking back on what I needed then and how I'm doing today, I think that if you don't need it, you are lucky. The less you depend on or *need* things, the better off you are! Having said that, we are snowflakes; we are different in our abilities so if your mobility remains compromised, then please use support. For me *now* it's just a walking stick as a support if I feel wobbly. That might have to stay a while.

Jaimee worked with me to strengthen my muscles, and to build endurance and stamina. I've learnt that it is important to get up and move around, *when you are able to*, and never without assistance first because of falls – so slowly does it. I eventually got to the point where I was riding the stationary bike for fifteen minutes, doing some arm exercises with weights, a few body combat moves with boxing and kicking; balancing on a soft surface, managing steps, and IMT exercises to keep my respiratory muscles in shape. I wasn't ready to run a marathon by this stage but I was doing very well. The exercises I was doing were just to get me to a baseline of mobility. From weak and wobbly I improved. It was just a matter of building on those gains every day.

I spent a lot of spare time walking around the unit and doing other exercises. It is up to each person to know what they can manage; all I can say is, do your best to get to a level of mobility that is good for you.

In MG it's best to exercise when you have the energy (meaning when you have rested, had your medication, and waited for 15–20 minutes before beginning your exercise). Pace yourself. Usually the morning is better, but as with most snowflakes the best time of day for exercise varies with each person. You have to tailor-make your own day when rehabilitating from a myasthenic crisis.

When exercising, you might do it in spurts: e.g. 15 minutes exercise, rest 3-5 minutes, 10 minutes exercise, rest, another 10 minutes exercise, rest and finish. You can repeat this throughout the day depending on your energy levels. Exercise serves as a way to keep the joints and muscles moving as they should. Exercising goals (if you have MG) are usually managing weight, maintaining a good level of mobility and strength, and looking after your health.

It's also important to know your own limitations and optimum times for self-care.

Some of the medication we take makes us put on weight. It increases the appetite, is fluid retentive, and stores fat around the body. While helping us it can initially exacerbate MG fatigue symptoms as well. So it's necessary to move around as much as you can and try to eat sensibly. It's really easy to just want to lie down and rest, because the fatigue you feel and the heaviness of your body makes you not want to exercise. It's a battle of will, and a balance that each one of us has to find between exercise and rest. There's a saying in the MG world: '*My get up and go wants to lay down and nap*'.

Back to my rehabilitation journey. I can say with confidence that by now I'm improving, I'm moving around independently, texting, and typing this story. Not so long ago my hands and fingers were so weak I couldn't text or hold the phone up, and my neck muscles couldn't hold my head up long enough to do any typing. I would say that most of this progress is due to the changes in medication and treatments prescribed by my neurologist. Now, I'm showering and doing things independently. I'm nearly at the end of my physio journey, because I am rehabilitating and doing very well, thanks also to the physiology input of Malcolm and Jaimee. I have come from hardly being able to move and having no strength, to being more independent with movement.

My ADLs (assisted daily living skills) and muscle strength in various different muscle groups has also improved.

♥

<u>August-September 2016</u>

Rehabilitation Ward STAR 2.

Mereti with Jess the
Ocupational Therapist.

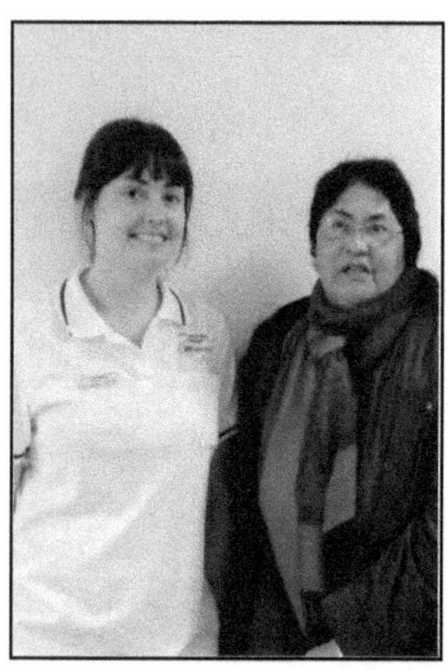

Telesia - Rehab. Social Worker.

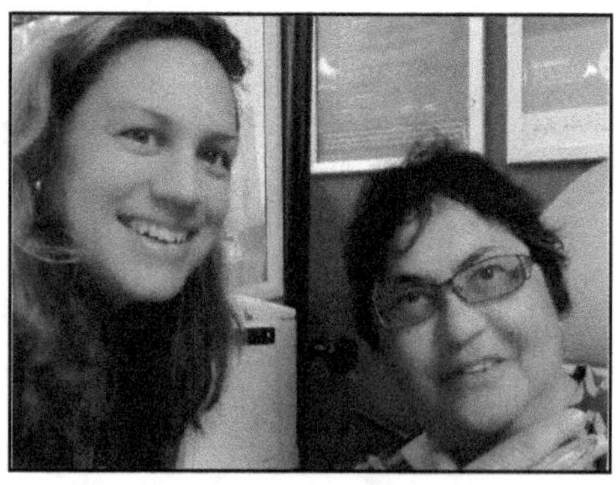

Chapter 18

Occupational Therapy

About two weeks into my stay in the rehabilitation ward, Occupational Therapy (OT) began. My Occupational Therapy Assistant was Cherine. At this time, I couldn't do much so Cherine helped me with ADLs, showering, grooming, and self-care. It was with her help that I got back to normal independence, to the point of being able to use a box shower like my one at home. I knew that by the time I was ready to go home, I would adapt very quickly. Cherine brought a kind, friendly, down to earth approach to her work, and she helped many of us in the ward.

We were all ages, with different abilities and levels of need, all of us wanting to get back to normal. The key messages I gained from our many talks were: to pace activities during the day, organise big activities like shopping and housework with someone to help, use the equipment that is offered, and make some lifestyle changes to help my wellbeing.

Occupational Therapy is a very interesting

field involving an eclectic cluster of work. It involves helping patients with everything from personal cares in the hospital, finding and providing alternatives for managing at home, setting routines to help with memory, providing equipment for safety, easy methods of cooking and following recipes, to managing workplace issues, and probably many things in between.

In the week beginning 29th August, Jess, the occupational therapist, contacted me to start planning kitchen ADLs, and equipment I might need at home. She had energy and wisdom, and for her young years, a lot of experience. She could see that it was now time for me to start working with Cherine in the kitchen: standing, motivation, energy levels, food choices, and efficient ways to cook. We would tackle shopping at the supermarket later – walking without assistance, standing for longer periods, and resting. The key message I gained from our talks was, again, to pace activities and do one main task a day: don't try to do lots of jobs at once, but organise them throughout the week. And ask family and friends for help when needed. Rest often, discuss what your needs are and the equipment you may need going forward.

Jess organised a visit to my home. This meant booking a vehicle, checking equipment and going to my house to carry out an assessment. Jess's assessment was spot on and invaluable with regard to the equipment and rails available. I still find these aids helpful. To this day I have incorporated what they taught me into my home life. Being at home more now, I use my spare time baking for visitors and family, and pacing my tasks so that I get everything done. I've learnt to ask for help from whānau and they, as usual, are always good to me.

♥

Chapter 19

Social Work

I'm sure that I was a little bit of a challenge when I first started to work with my social worker, Telesia Brown. I wasn't able to talk, I had a trachie in my throat and a nasogastric tube in my nose, so I was quite a sight, especially in the hospital gown and pants. And I was noisy and wobbly. But I knew what I wanted and Telesia was an easy person to talk to. Compassionate and without judgement, she brought life experience as well as a range of clinical skills to our work together and sorted out some of the jumble I was in. My first dilemma was the bank, and not being able to do my online banking. Telesia ended up having to contact the manager to negotiate a way around their red tape, and things seemed to start moving after that. Most of that dilemma was caused by the fact that I couldn't talk and just ring them to sort it out, and I couldn't go into the bank from the hospital as I had too many attachments and it was just too risky. Telesia did it though, and by the next week I was doing my online banking. She advocated on my behalf a few times so I could get help with anything I needed. She sorted out a medical alarm (and the payment for it), home help if I needed it, WINZ issues, and even getting the team together to focus on meetings or decisions that needed clarification. I was now able to leave the hospital confident that the things that I wanted in place, had been done. I had the St John's alarm installed, the home help was organised for six weeks, and I was able to do my banking and lots of other things, thanks to her work. Fa'afatai Lava e Telesia!

♥

September 2016
Rehabilitation Ward STAR 2.

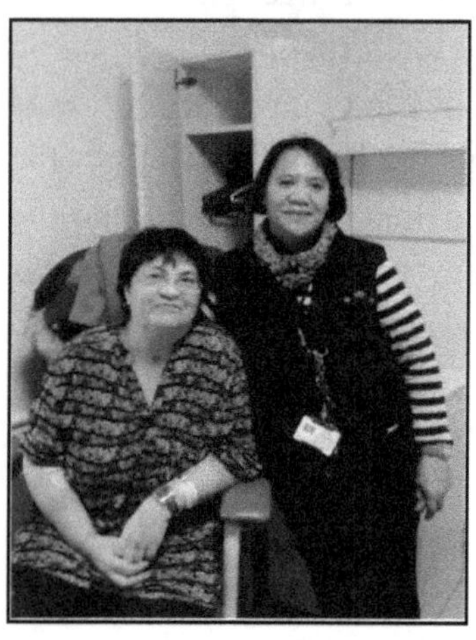

Mereti and Lorraine -
Mauri Ora facilitator
from Whare Rapuora.

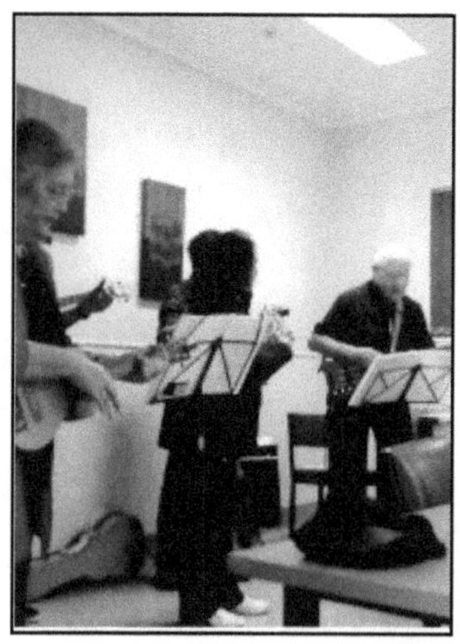

July 2016
Ukelele group from
Whare Rapuora
entertaining us in the
rehabilitation ward.

<u>May 2016</u>
Intensive Care Unit

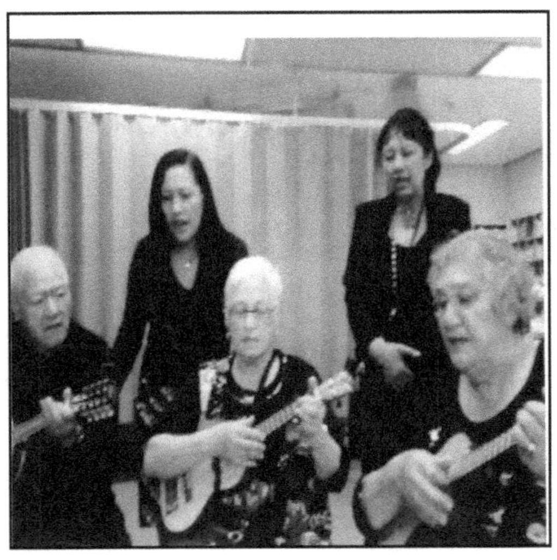

Ukelele group from Whare Rapuora

June 2016
Whare Rapuora

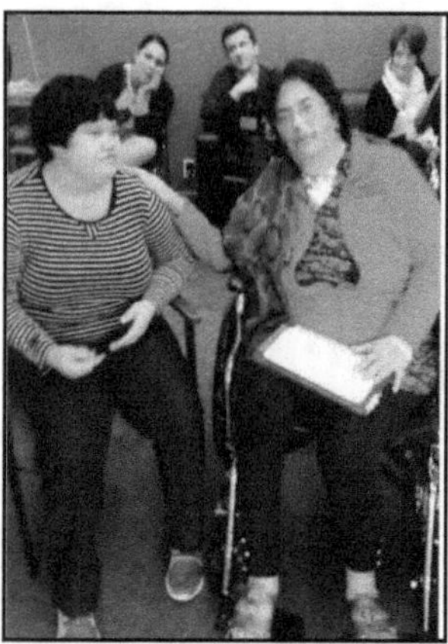

My daughter Ngaio and
I at Whare Rapuora

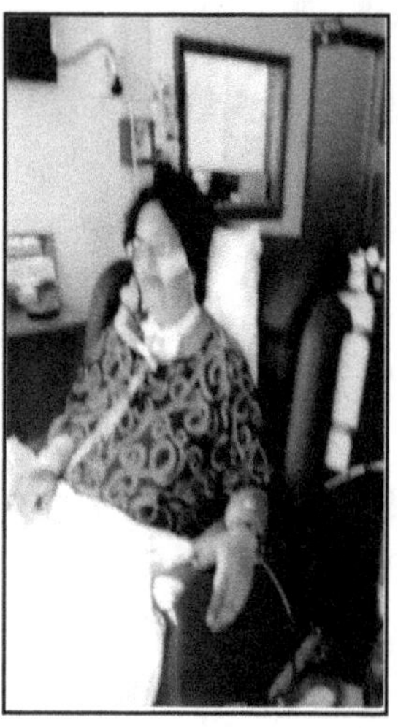

Connected to the mobile
ventilator and oxygen still.

Specialist Services within the hospital (2)

Chapter 20

Te Whare Rapuora

At this time I want to talk a little about Te Whare Rapuora, as I understand it. This unit is housed in a humble little whare that sits in the corner of the Hospital Grounds. For me, as a Maori patient and tangata whenua, the Whare Rapuora Unit means that the cultural needs of the tangata whenua are acknowledged and respected. Whare Rapuora staff provide cultural consultancy to the DHB, carrying out powhiri and other cultural protocols for all staff at the hospital.

Culture is important. New Zealand is now more culturally diverse than ever before.

Having said that, an important and unique benchmark in New Zealand's history (different from many other countries of the world), is that a treaty was entered into by the indigenous people (Maori or tangata whenua) and descendants of the British Crown. It was, and is, seen as a charter for the building of the three 'Ps' – Partnership, Participation and Protection, between the two signatories. The treaty is felt by many to be not only an historical contract but a *living* document. Whare Rapuora and the participation of cultural workers within the DHB is an acknowledgment of the three 'Ps' and of the treaty.

There are likely to be 'Whare Rapuoras' in other DHBs as well, all operating in a similar way to care for the whānau who visit their loved ones in hospital; to provide wairuatanga and to know and provide the correct protocols/tikanga for Maori patients, and to provide cultural consultation for the vast number of DHB staff.

To see the whare there and the whare workers within the hospital, is heartening for me and I'm sure many other Maori patients feel the same. I recall from my own contacts and knowledge of the Whare Rapuora that they have *both* cultural and clinical workers, spiritual minita-a-iwi and a roopu kaumatua who oversee processes of the whare. In line with the Mid-Central Health management, they have a manager and clerical workers. The chaplain, Tamati Pewhairangi, who is also a minita-a-iwi for the St Michaels Maori Pastorate, visited me regularly when I was very ill. He came to the ICU and carried out whakawatea, gave me karakia when I really needed and wanted it. Visiting me in rehab, he was a gentle presence, and I appreciated this.

Sometimes I wished Mum was there. In her sixties my mother trained and was ordained as an Anglican Minister. She became a minita-a-iwi (Maori Pastorate) working in the north for many years. When she returned home to the Manawatu, she was a minister for St Michaels church, Aorangi Marae, and then a hospital chaplain in Palmerston North Hospital. Her karakia were ngawari but powerful, and her presence so reassuring.

Looking back at my time in hospital, it was awesome that Tamati was there to spiritually care for me, and I know that Mum would be happy with that. When we are in such a dark place, karakia is a healing balm.

The Whare Rapuora is a fully staffed cultural unit that anyone can contact, and know that they will be welcomed. When the charge nurse from the ICU, Sue Kirkman, contacted the whare directly and talked to Lorraine Searancke (Mauriora Facilitator), it was from that conversation that everything was organised for my visit with my daughter. The collaboration of the ICU, the Whare Rapuora, and the staff who cared for my daughter, made it a success. What did being able to see my daughter do for me as a patient? It strengthened my resolve to get better. It also strengthened my wairua.

Those experiences, alongside clinical care, encouraged my recovery. Clinical care is the core business of any hospital for patient treatment and recovery, but this should not overshadow the importance of other types of healing systems. A person's wairua needs nurturing too; for many Maori patients it is grounding to address the spirit and to acknowledge the unseen.

The whare has workers throughout the hospital. Touching base with Maori people and helping them to feel comfortable while there is a wonderful thing. It's even better when people of other cultures can benefit from the feeling of manaakitanga, aroha, me te tumanako of the Kaiawhina Maori. The other aspect of Whare Rapuora is that it provides accommodation, and a home away from home (for a short while) for whānau that travel a long way to see their loved one in hospital. It provides respite for whānau wanting to rest, eat and relax after visiting their whānau member.

Te Whare Rapuora or the Maori Health Unit is your first port of call for Maori cultural services, and assistance for Maori patients. It is not an exclusive service (meaning anyone can see a Kaiawhina), but specialises in Maori service delivery.

♥

Part 3

Post-hospital Recovery

Chapter 21

Home Time

After being discharged from hospital on the 9th September 2016, it became more up to me how I coped at home. Most of the time I dealt with low-grade ongoing fatigue, and I found that some days were better than others. And … typical of MG, muscle weakness fluctuated constantly from day to day, and during the day, depending on what I did. If I did a lot of activity then I would need a lot of rest, and sometimes even if I didn't do much I needed to sleep a lot during the day. Another thing I am now aware of is that I have to do much more at home than when I was in hospital, so for a while I tended to get exhausted faster. Normally you wouldn't notice the extra things you do at home.

In the rehabilitation ward, the focus is on your strength, stamina, nutrition, mobility, re-learning things, and living skills. By the time you go home, you will be at a baseline of functioning independently. At home you will start to do more − like doing your own washing, walking further, showering yourself with no assistance, cooking, doing dishes, making your bed, putting out your rubbish, maybe feeding your pets, and so on. These are all extras, things you would've normally taken for granted. The advice of the specialists in the rehabilitation ward is invaluable in helping a person to make that transition. At home it's a work in progress; it's day by day until you recover.

The good side is that, even though it can take months, you can build your stamina and confidence by doing an activity every day, and that's what life is about: achieving something every day. I guess it's about your attitude to things; you've got to try and stay optimistic, and that is what will help you to get through each day until it becomes the norm once again.

I keep a journal, which I started in the rehabilitation ward with the occupational therapy assistant, Cherine, and I find that it helps keep me on track. It also helps me to keep tabs on what I have been doing, what my goals are for the day and what I've completed. The journal is also important for prompting my memory: I continue to improve by keeping active, both mentally and physically.

In my case (or in yours if you also have MG or a chronic illness), self-care is our own responsibility. I don't see myself as an invalid and I want to reclaim my independence, so as much as possible it's up to me to pave my way. It takes some positive thinking, sheer determination and a pinch of luck to do this. We are all different, but for me achieving my daily goals gets me through. It's feedback that allows me to tell myself, 'Yep, it's happening,' and 'Yep, Mum, I'm still here, and I'm OK.'

I've definitely adopted the 'Whare Tapa Wha' care model to guide me through. This is a Maori health model, and the philosophy of it has been around for centuries. But it was a very wise man (Sir Mason Durie) who developed it into a health model for use today, and one that is accessible to anyone. He gave it a name and outlined the elements of it. Whare Tapa Wha involves care of the physical, the mental health and aspirations, whānau and relationships, and the spiritual aspects of a person.

I think it is important to keep as fit as I can, so as my main form of dedicated exercise I walk, and use resistance bands when I have energy left. If I feel OK, and if I have the energy I may bake something to offer visitors, or I may do a little gardening; doing what I can every day is important to me. There is a saying that managers use and it goes like this:

'I can't do this, but I'm going to do it anyway,' – and I'm like that. The simplest of things can be quite daunting, but as they have to be done, you just do it. You have to resist talking yourself out of doing things.

Some days I have to spend a lot of time

resting and sleeping but it's par for the course. Now I know what to expect and I hope my experience helps you as well. The thing is, your body is just not going to be the same as it was, and you may have to adapt to a new 'normal'.

I also started the Green Prescription Programme and I found that very helpful in resetting me to life back in the community and accessing community services, like the gym. It helped me with regard to exercising and the importance of keeping that up, healthy diet, heart health, information on arthritis and diabetes, as well giving me the benefit of meeting others. At some points in your recovery you may have to ask for help; ask your family or friends for help if you need it. My son helped every weekend, and it would've been really hard at that time without any extra help with the heavier chores.

The latest event in my journey of recovery is that I have started the new treatment, Rituximab 1000mg: the first treatment was on Monday 5th December 2016. It was carried out in the oncology unit of the hospital and lasted for six hours. The long duration is necessary for the first treatment, because it gives your body time to adapt to the new infusion. I was given pre-medication first: saline, 100g methyl prednisone, Phenergan, then 1000g of Rituximab. My face swelled up like a ball due to the increased prednisone, and I slept most of the day because the Phenergan is a sedative as well as controlling any allergies that may arise. One of the concerning side effects, amongst others, is anaphylactic shock, so these pre-meds are absolutely necessary to enable the infusion to go as smoothly as possible. My next treatment is on the 19th December 2016.

♥

Chapter 22

Through my family's eyes

On the 10th of December, I was lucky enough to have a laid-back conversation with my thirty-year-old son, Tef, who has been looking after me and doing extras around home during the weekends. We always speak openly about things; everyone has their own view and it's important to acknowledge that, so there are no restrictions on what can be said. He's busy during the week but on some weekends he still comes out to give me a hand.

He vacuums, helps with laundry, housework, gardening and outside chores – now how many sons will do that for their mums, especially when he has things in his own life to manage? I'm a very lucky mum.

This is what he said when asked about my illness and hospitalisation:

'Well, I had to think about what had happened and change my game plan, and visualise my objective which was to be the man of the house. When it did

happen, and the thing that stays in my mind was when you had your cardiac arrest, I was frightened that you might leave this earth so to speak, or that you may not continue on as my mother, that certain things would happen if you were to pass away. I was frightened about (my sister) and how it would affect the family, holy damn, I did wonder what would happen. But by sheer chance my mother came back to this earth, you didn't pass away, you didn't leave us behind. I'm thankful for every day that you are alive and I'm thankful for being able to help out ... I want to let you know that you're important to me, and I know that you need me to step up and do my best to support the family. I need to take things more seriously now and face things with courage and sentience, and make my whānau proud of me.'

'What did you notice about the rest of the whānau, Tef? Your aunties and uncles?'

'What I noticed about them was, they were trying to be strong, expecting the worst but hoping for the best. We were trying to hash out the best option for you, looking at the 'what ifs' should you have passed away. We wanted it to be ... a time of celebration, of a life well lived, rather than our hearts pouring out blood and not being able to get through it. We wanted to acknowledge the life you lived and the things you tried to teach us, through tikanga

Maori or just doing things in your everyday life that were an example to us. But you came back, you ascended like a bird, like a phoenix from the ashes, you know? I don't know what the family thought, but I knew you would get through this.'

From talking to my siblings afterwards, I think what was going on in their minds was the thought that 'she could possibly die, because the doctors have just told us this', but in their hearts, they knew I wouldn't, knowing my fighting spirit and plain stubbornness, not to mention their refusal to believe it. In their hearts they knew I was very low, but that I would come back up again.

'Tef, how do you think I'm coping now that I'm at home?'

'I think you're coping pretty well, and you're learning more about the medications you have to take, which is really important. With this intelligence in mind, you'll learn to embrace new medical techniques, and learn more about the illness. This illness is something that people don't know a lot about and the medications you are on now, only regulate the current integrity of the disease. It will never go away, but it can be disabled in most of its parts.

'How do you think I am now, compared to how I was?'

'Oh, way better. A lot of what was harmful from the full effect of this illness, has not taken full effect on you, it hasn't taken everything from you, so I'm pretty pleased the way you've come back from it.'

My cousin Kathy visited me in hospital, offering foot massages, jokes, conversations. After a long day of sameness in the ward it was refreshing to hear of her latest escapades. It wasn't until a long time afterwards, when I returned home and she was helping me at home, that I asked if she would like to say something about how it was for her – and she said yes. With her consent I will share it with you:

'It's been a huge, very shocking experience, frightening, really frightening. I knew you were a strong woman but I've learnt even more just how stubborn and strong that you are. And you mentioned before, that stubbornness and your utter determination to survive. But also you were not just thinking about yourself, you were driven by your children, they were at your heart to get you through this. Why was it important to visit you in hospital? Well, we are cousins and I think of (your mum and my) Aunty, and we're family and that's what family does. When it comes to the crunch family just comes

out, and that's what's happened. I also thought of your children.'

'Had you heard of this condition before (MG)?'

'Well, yes, I found out about it, and it's been a few learning curves for me. It's a miracle sitting here with you actually, seeing that shine in your eyes, and seeing you laughing, and eating! I didn't think you would pull through, you know!'

'What did you think of the ventilator?'

'Well, you know I'm not new to this, having watched G (my husband) go through this, it brought back a lot of memories ... it made me think about things, but it is also what drives me, that if I can't come and visit, then it's selfish, and it's not about me, it's about the other person.'

'You saw me with all my attachments − do you think it would've been viable to have sent me home with the NGT and ventilator still attached?'

'One hundred percent, no way ... it horrifies me to think they'd even suggest it. That must've been hard for you, because you're not well, and you're weak, and you are having to stick up for yourself,

when they say to you, you will have to go home with the ventilator and NG tube in.'

'Thanks Kathy, you've got that right. I was weak, but in my mind I was determined I wasn't going to go home with all my attachments. I think I really dug my heels in at that time and decided I had to try harder to get better.'

I was also lucky enough to gain the perspective of one of my friends, Ngaire, who had been present when I first went into ED and who visited while I was in hospital.

She spoke about the time they first found out that I was ill and had to go to hospital:

'I was quite shocked, and it was a condition I'd never heard of, but I understood was quite rare, and it was a bit of a conundrum, because only a few weeks before we had been celebrating Mereti's 60th birthday, which my partner and I attended, and the next time I heard there was a short time in hospital and then she was in ICU. Later on my sister and I came down and she was still in the ICU, and she, uh, she had to have assistance with her breathing and couldn't communicate vocally, only with her eyes or her hands, and the whole situation was looking very, very grave. My sister just wanted to pray for Mereti. Neither of us are medical people, and just seeing her not being able to breathe or eat or speak was a shock.

122

My sister, all she could think of to do was to paint her toenails, but we felt there was nothing else, but a little personal touch – that's all we could do. A few months later, it was fantastic to hear that she had been transferred to the rehabilitation ward, but still not great. She had a hole in her throat and having to clean it out with suction. It was loud and you could see the mucus having to be sucked out of her throat. It just makes me think that there is a lot of indignities that happen for the patient. The medical profession takes it for granted (I notice), and there's no privacy. I just think as a personal and social experience for Mereti it was horrendous. All of Mereti's network which included her children, close family and friends ... all rendered helpless.

From Richard's (Ngaire's partner) perspective:

'I think he felt hopeless really, but he did his best with his visits and at least offered a friendly hand to hold. We felt much better when we knew she had been transferred to the rehabilitation ward.'

Yes – me too, I felt I had moved past the worst of it.

My younger brother, Tiratahi, is a man of few words but he helped me a lot by being there, from the time I had to go Wellington Hospital to the time I went to Palmerston North Hospital. During those times he kept an eye on things, and would transport me when I had day visits home, while at the same time living his own life. Like my other siblings, he knew I would get low, but that I would come back. My siblings know my stubborn nature my determined spirit, and although there were words of caution over my prognosis from doctors, they never swayed from their own thoughts.

My oldest brother, Charles, was there also throughout the whole ordeal; he was the point of contact for everyone – family, friends, colleagues and medical consultants. His job load was heavy, but as usual he stepped up and carried that mantle. He is also a man of few words, doing more than saying, making sure everything went well, and keeping a close eye on my care at the hospital. His comment was:

'I think what got you through was your stubbornness, but I knew it wasn't your time, even though I had been told by the consultant more than once. Do you know they told me more than once that they didn't think you were going to make it? I just thought to myself, nah ... she's strong, she'll be alright, she'll get through this ...'

'What was it like for you when I had the trachie in and couldn't talk?'

'It was terrible, it was hard to communicate and I found that hard. I couldn't understand what you wrote, at the time, because it was just one statement,' (he was wincing as he said this). *'It was frustrating.'*

My sister in law Sandy, said (jokingly):

'It was a pain, the midnight calls and not knowing what was happening and getting up to the hospital. One minute you were dying and the next minute you were awake and talking, and there was a time before, when I was visiting you in one of the wards and you broke into a sweat and I had to get the nurse, who came rushing in. I thought it was your heart. It was lucky I was there, as there was no one around, and that was the time not long before you had to have respiratory support.'

As I recovered my brother and sister in law were able to step back a little and take a breather. My oldest sister, Hurihia, who lives in another area, watched over my safety and recovery from afar by keeping in touch with our brothers. She visited when she could, and sent her sons to visit me when she couldn't come herself. She was involved for a long time and continues to keep in touch, making sure that I am doing well and keeping up with my appointments and daily goals. Some days when she visited, she would just sit with me all day and do her weaving while I slept. Or we'd just talk.

That's whānau. You don't always see them every day, but when the chips are down, they turn up and bolster you in their own ways, and sometimes we really need that support. I know I did.

♥

April - June 2016
Whānau visiting Mereti in the ICU.

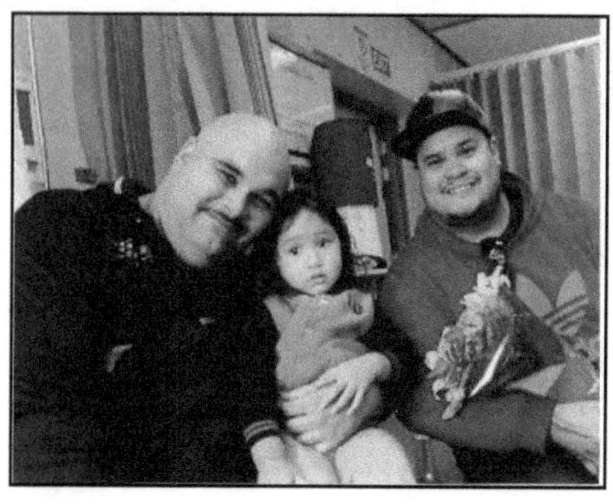

Nephews Puaha and Maha with Ake, Puaha's daughter.

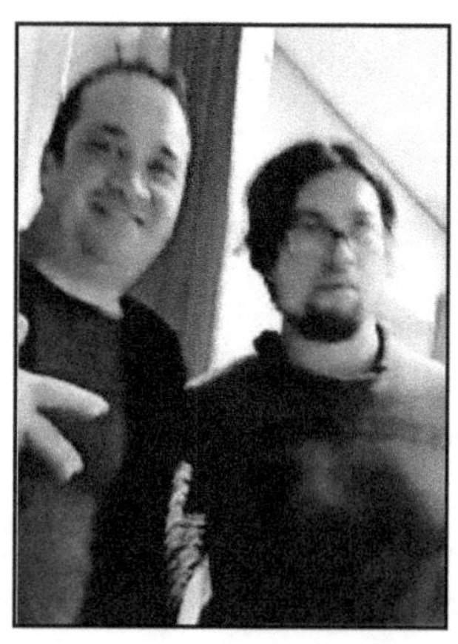

L-R Maui, youngest brother and my son Te Whiu.

March 2016

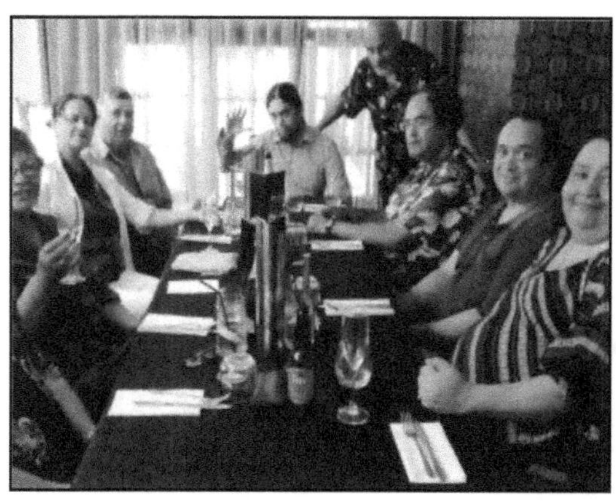

Whānau and friends out to a Birthday dinner.
L-R Mereti, Ngaire, Richard, Te Whiu, Charles,
Tiratahi, Maui, Shay.

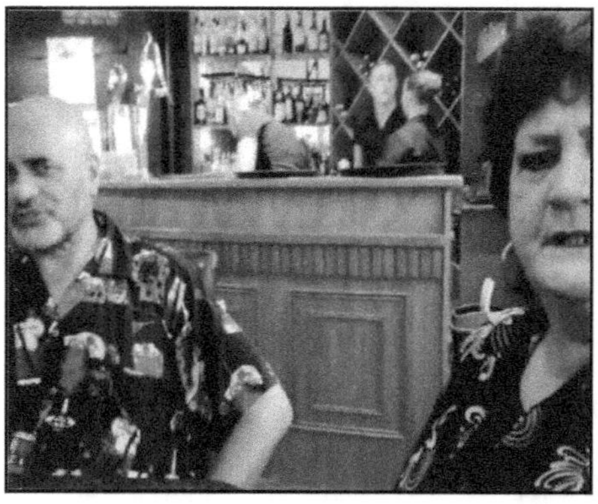

Brother Charles and sister-in-law Sandy.

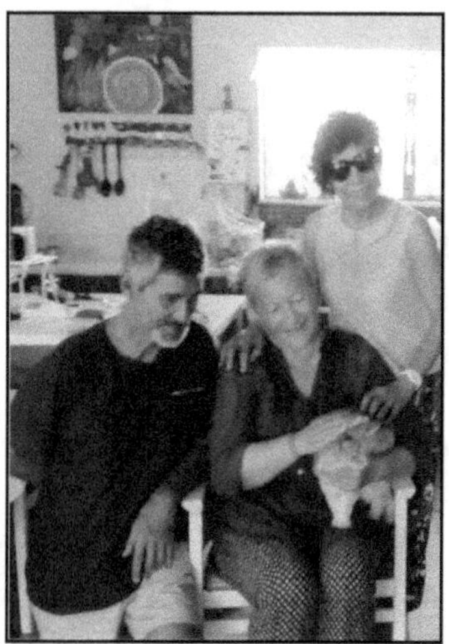

My cousins Rama, Ana and Kathy

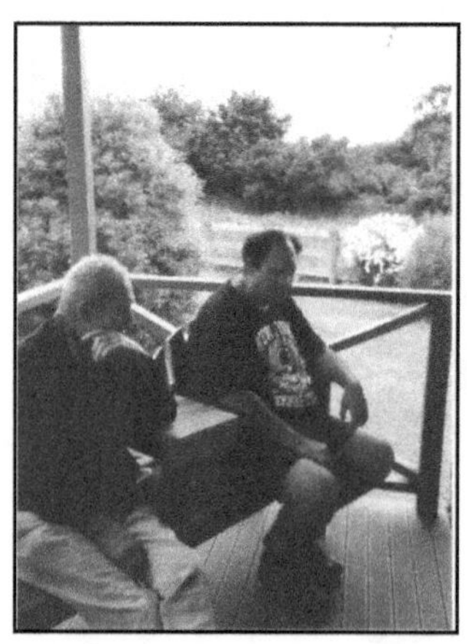

Whānau having a quiet chat.
Mason and Tiratahi

March 2017

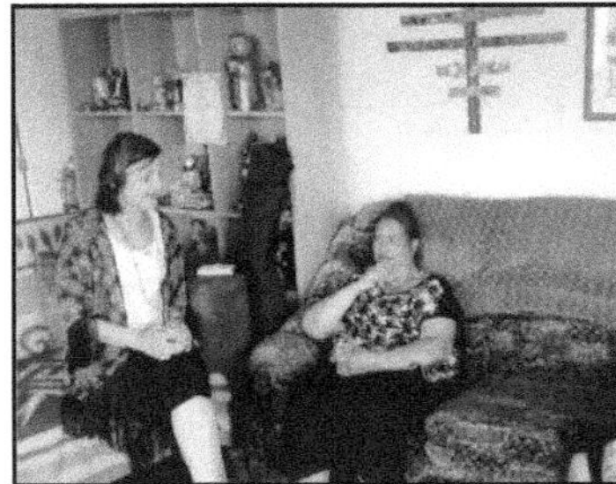

L-R Lea, Hurihia and Marcia.

Sandra and Raewyn from Totara Trust.

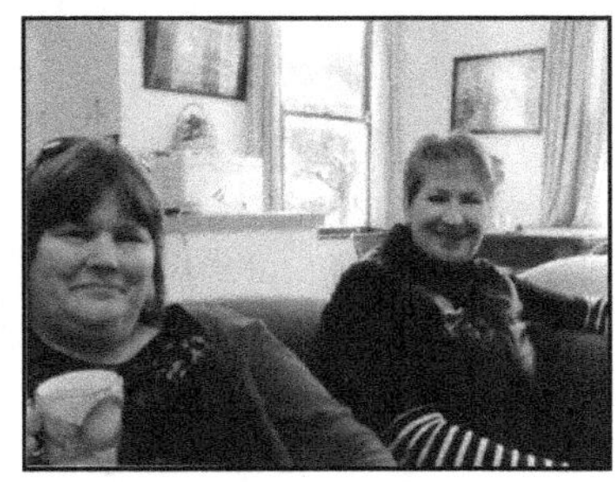

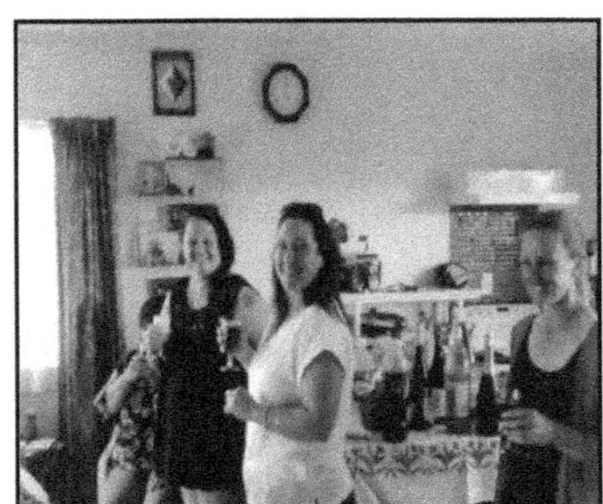

The girls from Totara Trust.
L-R Rachel, Sarah and Gabrielle.

<u>December 2016</u>

At Home

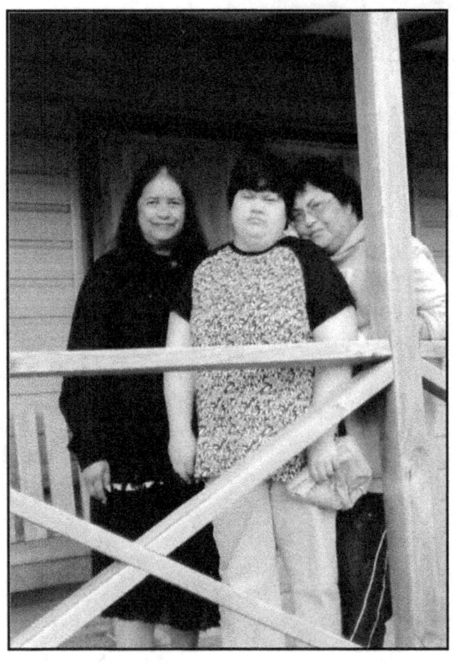

My sister Hurihia, Ngaio and I.
Home at last.

Chapter 23

The World outside My World.

There is a lot going on in the world today that may or may not affect us and our state of health. As this book is going to be a thing of the past one day, I thought I would include some notable things that happened this year (2016) in the world around me.

Leonard Cohen, the great singer and songwriter, died in November, and our own rockin' roller Ray Columbus died this month of December. On November 8th, Donald Trump was elected President of the United States, over Hillary Clinton. Now, this fact may affect access to healthcare, more so for MG sufferers in the United States. Previously there was Obama Care, or the Affordable Care Act, but if that is removed it will cause tremors throughout every community in the United States, as people scuttle to reassess their healthcare entitlements.

During the Trump presidential campaign one of the election promises was to repeal the Affordable Care Act. Without proper consultation with the American public and by just repealing the act without

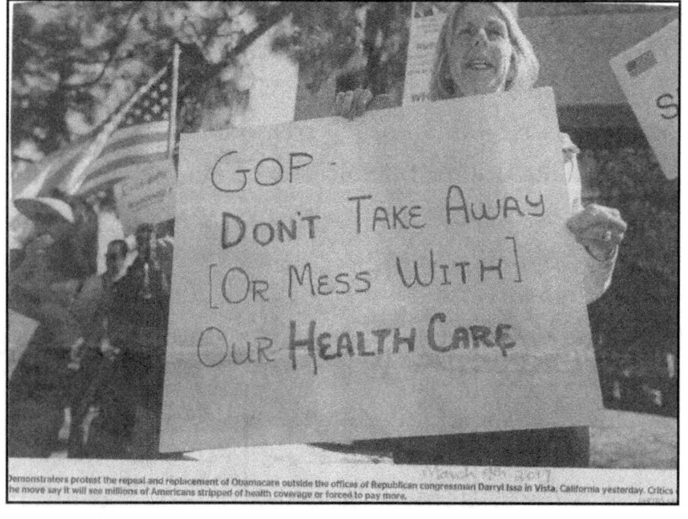

Demonstrators protest the repeal and replacement of Obamacare outside the offices of Republican congressman Darryl Issa in Vista, California yesterday. Critics of the move say it will see millions of Americans stripped of health coverage or forced to pay more.

analysing it, access to healthcare or healthcare insurance could be affected. This will impact on millions of people who are disabled by chronic illness or other conditions, may not be able to work, and therefore pay for health insurance without some sort of assistance.

I am a member of a few overseas website communities and at the time of writing this, there was a petition underway to gain public support for the RarePolicy.us. The Rare Diseases Policy would reinforce legislation of the treatment of rare diseases such as Myasthenia Gravis, and this is quite crucial as the USA health system is underpinned by health insurance. If one does not have health insurance, or any kind of bridging assistance that the Affordable Care Act offered for the majority of recipients, accessibility to healthcare and expensive treatments will be difficult.

Without the right healthcare, Myasthenia Gravis is still a terminal disease. This could happen in New Zealand should our free public healthcare cease and the government commodify health, allowing insurance companies to take over health and hospital care completely. Health care will then be something that can be manipulated.

The removal of the TPPA (Trans Pacific Partnership Alliance) trade deal due to USA withdrawal, may be a blessing in disguise for those with MG. Under the TPPA pharmaceutical companies may have had more control over prices, trade and distribution of pharmaceuticals.

John Key, our prime minister, announced his resignation on the 5th December 2016. He has named his successor to be Bill English. This change won't affect us in the short term, but it depends on who is

voted in as to how they will treat the population long-term, especially as there are those of us who, due to disability and illness, must depend on a benefit to live.

Under the National Government, the number of immigrants coming here and buying land and houses has increased and prices have skyrocketed. Without any kind of regulation on land and purchase of property by immigrants and foreigners, this will continue. This seems to show nothing but apathy towards the ordinary Kiwi citizen, as they are in effect being pushed out of the housing market. Their purchasing power is being nullified due to exorbitant house prices. There is not, as yet, any restriction on what off-shore or new immigrants can purchase; coming from larger, wealthier, longer established economies, the choices of what they can purchase seem endless.

The flow-on effect of that within NZ society is that the rich become richer, while the working class and those on low incomes, become marginalised. Unable to buy a house, perhaps even rent a house, the modest income earner becomes poorer.

There may be positives about increased immigration, but in 2017 these changes will not come about without impacting on our infrastructure. This includes our Health, Education, Cultural, Employment and Societal systems.

Many people with chronic illness, and disability, contribute to society by either working, volunteering, providing skills or labour. They make up about 5% of our population and provide employment for thousands nationwide in the caregiving, health and disability sectors.

Regardless of who the government of the day is, Health and Disability Policy should be robust and fair for all New Zealanders, and always include the views and input of those in the health, consumer and disability sectors. In that way we will remain a fairer, egalitarian society, resilient enough to meet the changes we are being faced with.

Summary

My MG crisis engaged many specialist services of the hospital such as the ICU, and Rehabilitation Ward Star 2 which included Physiotherapy, Occupational Therapy, Social Work, Transitionary Care Unit for IVIG, Oncology Unit for Rituximab, and the Speech Language Therapists. I learnt a lot from each of these specialist services – they were great. And I took home a lot of new knowledge about how to take care of myself. The support I received from whānau, friends, colleagues and others was amazing, and through that time of great uncertainty I couldn't have done so well without it.

At the last meeting with my neurologist, Dr Carigas, and Registrar Dr K Chang, we discussed other treatment possibilities. It looks like the Myasthenia Gravis is refractory, which means it is not responding to usual treatments, or is extremely slow to respond. This is where Rituximab or other treatments come in. Their use is unusual in New Zealand, but they had to use them for me.

While I am at this time making good progress, I am still at the tail end of the disease. The doctors also have a more defined diagnosis as to the type of MG I have: it is known as AChR, and is good in a way because treatment can be targeted. On the other hand, it's not good because it means the disease is further entrenched. The positive side is that I could still go into remission, which can happen with MG after a severe crisis and removal of thymus − so fingers crossed.

Going home was a transition of its own, and learning how to cope and look after myself was a mission as well, but I had the help of my son and occasionally other whānau members. Community home help agencies are very good, especially if there is no other person around to help. Recuperation time is the big unknown, so it's a wait and see game. So far it has taken a few months as it is now March 2017 and I was discharged on September 12th 2016. I'm still experiencing fluctuating symptoms, but as I am still at home and haven't had to go back to hospital, I am doing OK.

Things I have found helpful to me are: to keep a journal, attend Green Prescription meetings, exercise regularly, keep my house in order, have my family members and friends stay at times, rest frequently, and carry on − don't give up. I am looking at returning to work in April. When I think back that makes it about a year that I have been out of the loop with this illness.

A lot of time will be spent on building yourself up again, whether it's - carry on as usual, or a new normal, life goes on and there is always tomorrow.

<u>December 2016</u>

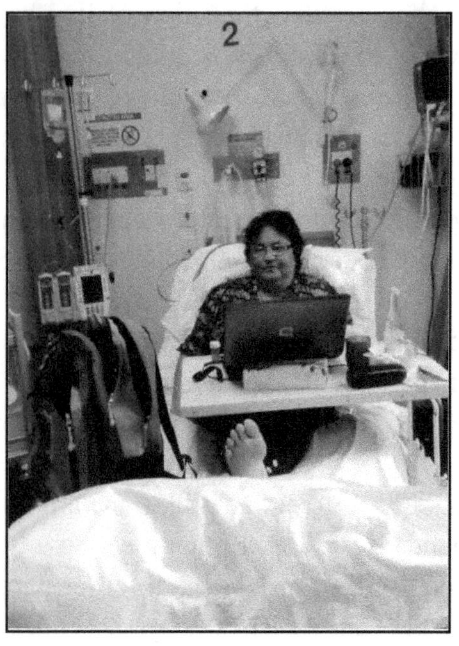

Having Rituximab treatment in the Oncology
Department at the hospital. I also have IVIG
treatments at the Transition care Unit 6 weekly.
Treatment after a major crisis is ongoing until
symptoms subside.

Epilogue

Ten things I have learnt from this experience:

1 **Whānau matter**
We are all part of a group, whether it be our kin, spouse, our friends, church or other group; this is our whānau and when the chips are down, it is so good to have them around. Whānau matter to us, and we matter to our whānau.

2 **Stubbornness + determination = endurance**
Throughout chronic illness, don't give up. It's a given that there will be pitfalls, but do what you can to stay focused until you get through it. There is a saying that goes like this: 'If you're going through hell, keep going.'

3 **The MG Dragon can be tamed**
Myasthenia Gravis is treatable, but it can be aggravated by other health procedures or illness. When the MG Dragon is aggravated, the weaponry required to conquer the Dragon's quest for death are the treatments, medication and knowledge of your consultants. This special medical weaponry can (and does) tame the MG Dragon.

4   Communication is key

Communication is a two way process. Medical professionals are there to help. Let them know what you need and work collaboratively with them. Don't assume that every doctor will know about this condition. Some of the communication skills you'll need are: assertiveness, patience, knowing how to inform others, listening and humour.

5   Treatment and care go together

Everyone feels apprehensive when they end up in hospital. It *is* about medication, equipment and treatments, but it's *also* about others (and self) and showing compassion for the person that is you.

6   Looking in and looking out (dealing with doubts by shifting the focus from the immediate situation)

It is tempting to get lost in MG and all the things that go with it. Although you need to know everything you can about the dragon, it is not your whole life. So look outwards to things beyond MG - what's happening at home, at work, with whānau, on the marae (or your community.)

7 Resilience can be learned
All I can say is, have faith in your own ability
to get through tough times. Life is about
meeting challenges, whether it's at home, at
work or in the hospital. If you can accept that,
then you're half way there. Create your own
'lifebuoy' to hold onto, until you can 'swim'
on your own − and you will.

8 Learning to live with some uncertainty
The MG Dragon will not leave you unscathed;
for a while you will continue to have
breathing and mobility problems, and muscle
weakness. There may be other health
procedures pending, or side effects from
medications.
Learning to live with uncertainty is part of the
territory.

9 There's no place like home
It's a strange feeling, but when you are in
hospital you miss your home, and when you
go home you miss the hospital. However if
you compare the white, sterile, shiny, beeping
surroundings with the multi-coloured, comfy,
cosiness that is your home, you know where
you would rather be. Once your treatment is
over, there really is no place like home.

10   **Getting on with it**

There are many community services that will
help you do just that! You just have to access
them and make it happen. Make use of
services like home help, Green Prescription
and other avenues. Have a plan every day, and
journal your progress.

The more you achieve, the better you feel and
the more you will be able to get on with it!

Tips for living the best life possible

MG symptoms can fluctuate

1. If you work, work part-time if you can. If you are symptomatic, you will then have time to recuperate.
2. It may be easier to exercise in 10-minute brackets about 3 times a day, when your medication is working at its best. You will know your own limitations.
3. Have bed rest when you can. Little power-naps are great for revitalising energy and give the body a chance to heal and recuperate.
4. Try not to enter into anything that could be too stressful. If you are symptomatic you will be vulnerable emotionally as well; it's just about your own self-care. Once again you will know your own limitations.
5. Keep a journal, and a graph to plot your own progress; this will also help you to recognise symptom improvements or worsening, and be a record of what you are able to do.

We need to be part of something

1. Stay in touch with others. Connection is important for our emotional wellbeing.
2. Friends and family are so important, to talk to,

for support, and for a soft place to land sometimes. Always keep the door open.

3. Be a part of an MG support group – local, national or international. Attend conferences if you are able to; get to know others and their story.

4. Maintain a balance between your physical, mental, spiritual and relational self. In New Zealand this is known as 'Te Whare Tapa Wha', a Maori model of wellbeing developed by Professor Mason Durie of Massey University.

5. Limit or eliminate anything that could be toxic to your system e.g: alcohol, tobacco, illegal drugs, pollution, and ongoing stress.

6. Cultivate your relationships, whether they are parental, friendships or a marriage partnership.

Taking care of your whole self

1. If you are working, be mindful of your work/life/family *balance*.

2. If you are not working, have a project you can do, whether it's painting, arts and crafts, or writing. A project will give you purpose and direction.

3. Be proud of yourself, know that you are doing the best you can even though you live with

MG. Self-esteem is important.

4. Keep a Gratitude Journal that you fill in every night. Answer the following:

>*Things I have achieved today
>*Ways I am lovable
>*People I am grateful for
>*Simple things that made me happy today
>*Things I couldn't do without

5. Meditate in a peaceful place, before the day starts or at the end of the day.

6. Visit Mother Nature often: parks, beaches, the bush, rivers or just your garden. Nature promotes harmony, feel-good endorphins and grounding.

Evacuation Plan

Have an evacuation plan written down and discuss it. These are times of climate change and times of flood, earthquake, and high winds. In case of fire, we will need to get to a safe place, without running out of breath, being too fatigued, or falling. So how will you mobilise? How will you keep in touch with everyone (if there are no cell phones)?

And remember your emergency kit.

<u>2017</u>
Walking towards a 'new normal'.

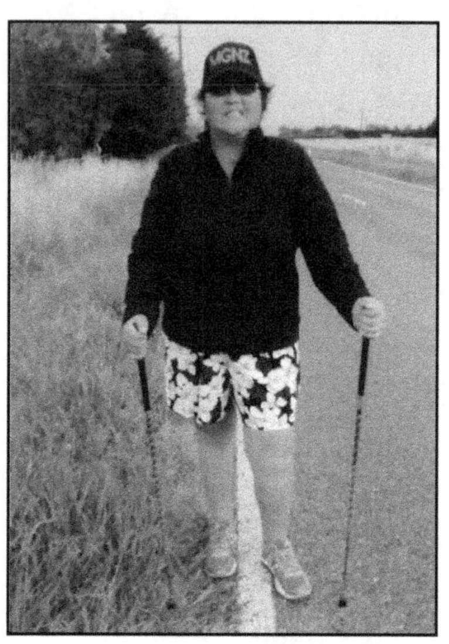

<u>He Whakatauki Maori: A Maori Proverb</u>

Mauri ora ki te atua
Mauri ora ki te whenua
Mauri ora ki nga tangata
Mauri ora kia tatou katoa

Blessings to god and the spiritual
Blessings to the land we live on
Blessings to mankind and care of this earth
Blessings to us and all people everywhere.

RESOURCES AND CONTACTS

Mereti Taipana-Howe (2016) Author of
Taming the MG Dragon: Journey through a Myasthenic Crisis
Myasthenia Gravis, an autoimmune disease
e: mereti2004@inspire.net.nz
https://www.facebook.com/snowflakesanddragons

An App that you can download onto your phone:
MyMG = search Google and download. Contains a variety of information about MG, and mini-lectures from neurologists who specialise in MG treatments.

New Zealand Myasthenia Gravis Support Group (NZMG)
Contact person: Talitha Vandenberg
Ph: 0272203138
Pahiatua

Muscular Dystrophy Organisation – is the National umbrella organisation for neuromuscular disorders which includes Myasthenia Gravis.
Contacts: Free Ph: 0800 800 337 - all regions
Ph: 09 8157260
PO Box 12063
Penrose, Auckland

148
Contact: Heather Browning, Chairperson

There are also Fieldworkers who cover different regions.

Books by people who have Myasthenia Gravis:

Putnam-Hill, Teresa; (2012) *The Show must go on: Overcoming Obstacles through positive thinking.* Charleston, USA.

Vandenberg, Talitha (2016) *My mummy has Myasthenia Gravis,* Palmerston North, New Zealand.

Other Book sources:
Durie, M.H. (2001) Mauri Ora: *The dynamics of Maori Health* pp; 173,174, 237-239, 238, 241-243.(Whare Tapa Wha) Oxford, New York

Websites sources:

*http://www.myasthenia.org.au

* http://www.myasthenia.org

                                                                    *
https://www.facebook.com/SupportMyastheniaGravis

* *emedicine*.medscape.com

* *www.nzord.org.nz/support_groups*

* http://www.livestrong.com/article/477048-physical-therapy-for-myasthenia-gravis/

*http://www.myasthenia.org/LinkClick.aspx?fileticket=VGYZpqsdfdE%3D&tabid=125#page=1&zoom=auto,-98,797

(Topic: The Neurologist : Myasthenia Gravis, January 2002, Volume 8, Number (1)

 * http://www.dailystrength.org/group/myasthenia-gravis/discussion/bladder-and-bowel-problems

* http://lisadouthit.com/the-top-dos-when-living-with-an-autoimmune-disease

* http:// www.myastheniagravis.org

Websites of interest

* https://www.nursingtimes.net/clinical-archive/gastroenterology/nasogastric-tubes-2-risks-and-guidance-on-avoiding-and-dealing-with-complications/5000684.article
*

150

http://www.hopkinsmedicine.org/tracheostomy/about/how.html

* http://www.livestrong.com/article/477048-physical-therapy-for-myasthenia-gravis/

*

https://www.google.co.nz/?gws_rd=ssl#q=what+happens+after+trach+is+removed

*

https://sites.google.com/site/studentcapstone100/home/mg-occupational-therapy/ot-intervention

* https://www.stgeorges.nhs.uk/gps-and-clinicians/clinical-resources/tracheostomy-guidelines/post-decannulation/

*

https://sites.google.com/site/studentcapstone100/home/mg-occupational-therapy/ot-intervention
146
https://www.youtube.com/watch?v=QC4uYYo171k
* http://www.sca-aware.org/sudden-cardiac-arrest-faqs

There are also a lot of medical websites available to the health sector.

Hospital contacts for Maori clients

Te Whare Rapuora (Maori Health Unit)
Palmerston North Hospital

GLOSSARY

Maori to English

Aroha	Compassion
Fa'afatai Lava	Thank you (Samoan)
Hapori	Your community
Kaiawhina/kaimahi	Maori worker
Karakia	Spiritual blessing/healing
Mahi	Your work/contribution to others
Manaakitanga	Care for others
Marae	Tribal meeting place
Mauriora	Wellbeing
Minita-a-iwi	An ordained minister with the Maori Pastorate
Mirimiri	Massage
Nga piki me nga heke	Ups and downs
Ngawari	Gentle
Pou	Strength
Powhiri	Formal welcoming ritual
Tangata Whenua	Indigenous people of Aotearoa/Maori
Tikanga	Protocols/Way things are done
Tumanako	Hope
Wairua	Spirituality
Whakawatea	Spiritual clearing

Whānau	Small and extended family (sometimes used to denote belonging to a group). Family members
Whānau whanui	Wider whānau, all related
Whare	House/building

Medical Abbreviations

ACH-R	Category of Myasthenia Gravis
ADLS	Assistance in Daily Living Skills
Airvo	Airflow tubes placed in the nose to help keep lungs inflated
BiPAP	Bivalve breathing mask
CPAP	Breathing Mask
CPR	Cardio Pulmonary Resuscitation
DHB	District Health Board
ENT	Ear Nose and Throat
FEES	Fibre optic Endoscopic Evaluation of Swallowing (Speech Language Therapy Dept)
ICU	Intensive Care Unit
IMT	Inspiratory Muscle Trainer for strengthening respiratory muscles
In situ	In the site (of the operation or procedure)

IVIG	Intravenous Immunoglobulin treatment for MG
MDT	Multiple Disciplinary Team
MG	Myasthenia Gravis
MG Dragon	Life threatening crisis, lasting longer than a month where mechanical ventilation is required to breathe.
MUSK	Category of Myasthenia Gravis
Nebs	Saline Nebuliser
NGT	Nasogastric Tube
OTA	Occupational Therapy Assistant
OT	Occupational Therapy/Therapist
Physio	Physiotherapists

Respiratory muscles

The muscles that produce volume changes of the thorax during breathing. The inspiratory muscles include the hemidiaphragms, external intercostals, scaleni, sternomastoids, trapezius, pectoralis major, pectoralis minor, subclavius, latissimus

156

dorsi, serratus anterior, and muscles that extend the back. The expiratory muscles are the internal intercostals, the abdominals, and the muscles that flex the back

Snowflake Nickname given to people diagnosed with Myasthenia Gravis

SLT Speech Language Therapy/Therapists

Trachie (1) Tracheotomy - an incision in the throat to enable breathing the placement of a tracheostomy.

Trachie (2) Tracheostomy - is the tube that is placed in the throat incision. which enables attachment to a ventilator to assist breathing. It also enables breathing without a ventilator, and prevents aspiration.

VHSS Video fluoroscopic Swallowing Study (Speech Language Therapy Dept)

Hospital Terminology

Aspiration

Choking as food or water goes down the windpipe due to swallowing difficulties (weakness of bulbar, or oesophageal muscles)

Consultants

Senior specialists in their field

Decannulation cannula

Removal of tracheotomy, or

Endotracheal tube

This is also called an ET tube. It is put into your mouth or nose to keep your airway open. It may be attached to a ventilator to help you breathe, and you may get extra oxygen through your ET tube. You will not be able to talk while the ET tube is in place.

Intravenous Immunoglobulin (IVIG)

An infusion to treat Myasthenia over 4 - 6 hours

Intubation

When a breathing tube is placed in the throat of a patient to enable regular breathing. Also

	installation of NGT.
Junior Doctors	Graduate doctors, internship training
Lip sealing exercises	SLT exercises to strengthen the lips and cheeks, to help with speech and controlling the mouth for eating, swallowing etc.
Oromotor	SLT exercises to get the mouth, cheek, tongue muscles working.
Oesophageal	Of the oesophagus (food pipe)
Plasmapheresis	A treatment for Myasthenia Gravis, used in crisis or to prevent one.
Registrars	Doctors training in a specialist field.
Rituximab	A new treatment for MG ACH-R. or Rituxin.Still undergoing clinical trials, but also being used in some countries around the world where there are no

other effective treatments.

Ventilator	Breathing machine, necessary
when MG compromises respiratory

Yankauer	Part of tracheotomy care, to
suction saliva away because patient's
swallowing and oesophageal muscles
are not working.

Myasthenia Gravis Clinical Terminology

Acetylcholine

A chemical released by a nerve ending that activates a muscle cell to contract and generate force.

Acetylcholine receptor

A protein substance on the muscle cell membrane which accepts acetylcholine from the nerve ending.

Acetylcholine receptor antibody test

A blood test for these abnormal antibodies which can be performed to see if they are present. Approximately 85% of MG patients have this antibody and, when detected, is a guaranteed diagnosis.

Acetylcholinesterase

An enzyme located in the gap between a nerve ending and the muscle cell membrane whose function is to inactivate acetylcholine

Anti-MuSK antibody test

A blood test for patients who have tested negative for acetylcholine antibodies. Of these, 40% to 70% test positive for the anti-MuSK antibody. The remaining patients may have an antibody to LRP4 or an unidentified antibody causing their MG.

Autoimmune disease

A disorder caused when the body fails to recognize

itself and mounts an immune attack (usually reserved for invading bacteria or viral infections) producing antibodies against its own tissue. In MG, the acetylcholine receptors are the victims of this misdirected immune attack.

Bulbar MG

Myasthenic weakness involving the muscles for speech, chewing and swallowing. The name derives from the fact that the nerve supply to those structures comes from the medulla or "bulb" of the lower brain.

Corticosteroids (steroids)

Hormones used to dampen the faulty immune response that occurs with MG.

Crisis

A term for "acute respiratory insufficiency" developing over hours or days and severe enough to require assisted mechanical support for breathing. Usually, the respiratory insufficiency is the result of weakness of the diaphragm and intercostal (rib) muscles, but it also can occur if weak throat muscles obstruct the airway.

Diplopia

The perception of two images in the field of vision. Ocular myasthenia may affect the eye movements in vertical, horizontal, or diagonal directions, with variable degrees of double vision.

Dysarthria

Difficulty speaking, producing slurred, breathy words which are poorly understood. It results from weakness of the muscles used for speech.

Dysphagia

Difficulty or inability to swallow.

Generalized MG

MG affecting more than just the eye muscles (contrasted with pure ocular MG).

Hyperplasia of the thymus

When the number of thymus cells increases and the thymus becomes enlarged.

Immunosuppressant drugs

Medications which modulate or suppress the body's immune system, to hopefully reduce symptoms of an autoimmune disease. In MG, a reduction of circulating acetylcholine receptor antibodies may improve strength.

Intravenous Immune Globulin (IVIg)

An expensive medical procedure involving intravenous infusion of human gamma globulin antibodies pooled from multiple donors, which results in rapid but temporary relief of MG symptoms.

MuSK

Patients without serum antibodies to acetylcholine receptor (seronegative MG) may instead have antibodies to muscle-specific kinase (MuSK), another protein at the neuromuscular junction.

Neonatal myasthenia

Myasthenic weakness lasting two to twelve weeks in a newborn infant as the result of a passive transfer of acetylcholine receptor antibodies from the mother.

Neuromuscular

Nerves and muscles.

Ocular myasthenia

An autoimmune condition characterized by variable weakness of the muscles of the eyelids and eye movements. This leads to droopy eyelids (ptosis), double vision (diplopia), or both.

Plasmapheresis

Also called "plasma exchange." An expensive medical procedure that separates the blood into its two major components: plasma (the liquid part of the blood) and cells. The blood cells are then returned to the patient, with the plasma being replaced by a blood product called albumin or a plasma substitute. Performed by a machine similar to that used for kidney dialysis.

Ptosis

Droopiness of eyelids caused by muscle weakness. In ocular myasthenia, ptosis is usually variable and worsens as the day progresses.

Seronegative MG

Myasthenia gravis that is clinically suspected in patients even though blood tests for the acetylcholine antibody or MuSK antibody are negative.

Skeletal muscles

Any muscle you can move by thinking about it.

Thymoma

Tumour of the thymus gland.

Thymus

A flat, H-shaped gland lying mainly behind the breastbone (sternum) and in front of the heart. It is important for immune system development early in life, and shrinks with aging.